Recognizing spiritual needs in people who are dying

Rachel Stanworth

Former Researcher at St Christopher's Hospice, London
Management Advisory Committee member and trainer for The Befriending Network, London

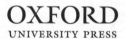

OXFORD
UNIVERSITY PRESS

OXFORD
UNIVERSITY PRESS

Great Clarendon Street, Oxford OX2 6DP

Oxford University Press is a department of the University of Oxford.
It furthers the University's objective of excellence in research, scholarship,
and education by publishing worldwide in

Oxford New York

Auckland Bangkok Buenos Aires Cape Town Chennai
Dar es Salaam Delhi Hong Kong Istanbul Karachi Kolkata
Kuala Lumpur Madrid Melbourne Mexico City Mumbai Nairobi
São Paulo Shanghai Taipei Tokyo Toronto

Oxford is a registered trade mark of Oxford University Press
in the UK and in certain other countries

Published in the United States
by Oxford University Press Inc., New York

A catalogue for this title is available from
the British Library

ISBN 0-19-852511-7 (Pbk)

10 9 8 7 6 5 4 3 2 1

Typeset by EXPO Holdings, Malaysia
Printed in Great Britain
on acid-free paper by Biddles Ltd, Guildford & King's Lynn

Foreword

Dame Cicely Saunders, OM, DBE, FRCP,
Founder/President St Christopher's Hospice

'There is no deeper longing, and no wish more suited to the contemporary
scene, than the longing to recognize and be recognized, the longing for
fulfilment through recognition' (Harper 1955). The numerous illustrations,
given by patients' comments as they tell their story, make this book a truly fascinating journey through an important area of end-of-life care. This contribution to a facet of care more often acknowledged than carried out with any
confidence is the result of a study completed after wide reading and with a
personal sensitivity. Someone to whom a patient with motor neurone disease
types 'I am me at last, free to be my own silly self' and also that she is 'stepping
out of an unhappy place into a freedom to develop my own feelings and attitudes' is listening to responses given in a gentle and deep attention. This
patient finally writes 'my hope is that it [the illness] will lead me into peaceful
waters, sailing on a calm sea. I have expended so much anger in the past and
have longed to get rid of it. It seems that this tragedy has taken me on that
path at last.' She is using the language of the spirit in an acknowledgement of
this personal recognition. Such comments reveal how the writer has achieved
her purpose of discovering spiritually significant patterns of meaning and
perceptions of selfhood. Her meetings have truly brought the affirmation so
often lacking at the end of life.

Twenty-five patients in St Christopher's Hospice were asked to take part in
the study. They were introduced by a member of the ward or homecare team
to the researcher. Rachel Stanworth used a tape recorder because, as she said
'I'm interested in how you see things—what's it like for you.' This quiet
encouragement to tell a personal story was rewarded. Throughout the exploration, carried out without techniques or questionnaires, profound theological
and psychological insights are continually grounded in the responses of
people obviously at ease with an enabling listener.

Metaphors were constantly employed by the 25 interviewees, many of
whom had little or no religious background or language. The writer of the
'calm sea' and another patient, the owner of the dying flowers kept on
her locker because, as they set seed, they spoke to her of new life, are such

examples. Stanworth also sees them as sources of meaning revealed and constructed in a fascinating key diagram. This exploration prepared her listening and enlightened her subsequent discussion. As she writes, 'metaphors give access to depths otherwise inaccessible. Science, religion and the arts all rely on this.' Expressing this in a symbolic form, she addresses the whole person, not just the intellect.

Such listening and meditation is costly. Stanworth gives a perceptive list of helpful guidance to those who embark on such a quest but is also encouraging for those who have many other tasks to fulfil and may be daunted by her unhurried recognition of such insights. The time available to pastoral workers and other staff may be very varied and we must never forget that 'the way care is given can reach the most hidden places and give space for new development' (Saunders 1996). Stanworth writes of the patient who found a nurse's presentation of a cool pillow to her as her most effective spiritual help and of the incontinent man who found that a blanket bath, during which he was gently included in conversation, restored him to his sense of self. As he said, 'in the end, you don't give a damn' as all his 'silly male pride' evaporated. Stanworth notes 'Those who wish to respond with sensitivity to the total needs of a dying person are not called on to resolve doctrinal issues or to make dogmatic statements but to realise their own wholeness as far and as authentically as they can.' Persevering with the practical is an important step along this discovery.

Time in palliative care is so often a matter of depth rather than length. Those who have to hurry on to meet the needs of the next patient and family can be stimulated here to use the time available in a moment of true attention. Although she did not interview their families, Stanworth met young women struggling to come to terms with handing over the care of their children to others. One family made a 'statue' of their mother in a corner of their home and a photograph of this poignant image is included. After discussing it at great length, the mother was able to say 'They'll know when its time to put it away.' This photograph and the series of paintings by another patient, who had said 'You can't leave earth with a grudge' add much to the profound message of this book. Its perspective is that of pastoral theology but its message is a quiet challenge to the humanity we share with those we care for. As Stanworth writes 'Spiritual care is like a good story, demanding a response from the whole person.'

This is not a book giving techniques or suggestions for making a spiritual profile, rather it presents a project of qualitative research giving insights for which we should be very grateful. Patients' words are afforded their full dignity of meaning and it shows how a group of people revealed their own potential for exploring the depths of what it can mean to be human. As Stanworth says 'The most important thing I brought to the interviews was not my questions but my silence.' The space that silence gave was filled with individual searches for meaning and fulfilment at a level that should challenge our living as well as our practice, for it is 'not what we know but how we are with patients that makes all the difference to their care.'

References

Harper, R. (1955). *The sleeping beauty.* Harper and Brothers, New York.
Saunders, C. (1996). Foreword to Kearney, M. (1996). *Mortally wounded.* Marino, Dublin.

Acknowledgements

I am extremely grateful to the Sir Halley Stewart Trust for funding my position as Chaplaincy Researcher at St. Christopher's Hospice for three years. The kind assistance of The Society of Authors has also been instrumental in allowing me time to write. Beyond any financial assistance, however, I am indebted to Rev. Len Lunn my manager at St. Christopher's for his unfailing support and encouragement, as well as to numerous other colleagues for their insights and experience. I also owe an immense debt of gratitude to my academic supervisor Dr. F. J. Laishley. The advice and guidance of Catherine Barnes and Kate Smith, my comissioning and production editors, is gratefully acknowledged along with my conversations with Josefine Speyer, Dorothy Watson, Terry Salerno, and many people involved with the Befriending Network, an organization that links carefully selected and trained volunteers with people who are living with a life-threatening illness.

I am mindful that Dame Cicely Saunders' characteristically thoughtful foreword is a tremendous honour and I am very grateful. I also want to thank those relatives who have kindly given me permission to reproduce their loved one's art and to publish the photograph of Tracey's 'statue'. Even beyond the appreciation extended to my forbearing husband and family, however, lies my gratitude to those patients who so generously made this book possible and to whose memory it is dedicated.

Preface

When St Christopher's Hospice in South London, in conjunction with
Heythrop College, University of London, advertised for someone to conduct a
piece of doctoral research into any aspect of the spiritual needs of terminally
ill people, I applied. My existential curiosity had been aroused by several years
spent nursing, working for a disability charity and later helping to develop a
befriending scheme for people diagnosed with a life-threatening illness. When
family and professionals have made every effort to alleviate suffering and all
avenues of support have been exhausted, I wanted to know where a dying person can 'stand' when it seems there is no ground underfoot and when all of
life's familiar landmarks have shifted. Are there satisfactory answers to radical
questions such as, 'Why me?' or, 'Why now?' How do people find them?
Beyond the limits broached by medicine, psychology or the humanities is
there a further and all-encompassing horizon that gives meaning to human
life and its finitude?

This book explores these and other questions from the 'inside' in that everything it says is grounded in the words and experiences of terminally ill people.
After listening carefully to the stories of 25 hospice patients and conducting a
period of participant observation on one of the wards at St Christopher's, I
have tried to construct a new story that shows something of human spirituality and the experience of facing death. Hopefully, this showing does not distort
or misrepresent the original narratives but will augment current thinking on
spirituality in palliative care and advance the insight, confidence and compassion of readers by encouraging them to reflect on their own relations with
seriously ill people.

Rachel Stanworth
2003

Illustrations

Fig. 3.1 Distributions of participants by gender. (Colour Plate 1.)
Fig. 3.2 Distribution of participants by age and by gender. (Colour Plate 2.)
Fig. 6.1 Sources of meaning and sense of self in people who are dying (revealed and constructed by metaphor).
Fig. 7.1 Vase of dried flowers. (Colour Plate 3.)
Fig. 7.2 On the beach. (Colour Plate 4.)
Fig. 9.1 Sewing woman. (Colour Plate 5.)
Fig. 9.2 On the balcony. (Colour Plate 6.)
Fig. 11.1 Tracey's statue. (Colour Plate 7.)
Fig. 12.1 Reclining nude. (Colour Plate 8.)
Fig. 12.2 Carla's bride. (Colour Plate 9.)

Contents

Glossary

Anamnesis Greek for the recalling of things past. A process of learning akin to recognition that accounts for our understanding of events or types of knowledge that we have not previously consciously experienced or studied.

Anima mundi Latin for 'world-soul'. The universe is regarded as endowed with a soul or spirit by a supreme power or creator to ensure its harmonious workings.

Archaic A word or language no longer in ordinary use, although employed for special purposes, as in ceremonial situations or in poetry. Also resorted to by individuals who are experiencing acute stress.

Archetype Although culturally variable, archetypes are common to all people and express the identity and continuity of man's psychic structure. They are not experienced directly but through the medium of symbols, taking various forms and personages such as those of the archetypal mother or trickster or a range of mythological figures.

Collective unconscious Psychic material not immediately available to consciousness but common to all people or shared by particular groups of people.

Connotative When, in addition to any possible literal or primary meaning, particular words or deeds have the quality of suggesting other associations or ideas.

Denotative Having the quality of denoting, designating or pointing to specific or existing objects of reference.

Eschatological Pertaining to the final destiny of individuals and humanity.

Etymology The process of tracing the history of words and accounting for their formation, development and meaning.

Existential Pertaining or relating to the conditions of human existence

Hermeneutics Pertaining or relating to theories of interpretation.

Liminality From the Latin for threshold. Pertaining to a sense of transition, of feeling neither 'here' nor 'there'.

Metanoia From the Greek for changing one's mind. A re-orientation of one's life. Often used to describe a spiritual or religious conversion.

Metaphor To speak of one thing in terms that are suggestive of another thereby disclosing and creating realms of meaning that previously escaped observation.

Metaphysics A matter of asking questions concerning matters that are not empirically verifiable.

Ontology Pertaining or relating to the nature or essence of being or existence.

Palliative care An approach that improves the quality of life of patients and their families/significant others facing the problems associated with life-threatening illness, through the prevention and relief of suffering by means of early identification, assessment, and treatment of pain and other problems: physical, psychosocial, and spiritual. This 'total care' is characterized by a multi-disciplinary team approach.

Platonism Refers to the ideas of Plato, particularly those relating to his theory of forms or ideas: the concept of logical and/or mathematical entities having an untainted existence that is independent of both human thought and the empirical world.

Po(i)esis Greek. Any imaginative use of language that both discloses and mediates hitherto unsuspected aspects of reality.

Religion The life complex of practices, norms and structures of a community, which find their origin in a founding revelation.

Spirituality The interpretative story and ensuing values of an experience that is regarded as both human and ultimate. Not necessarily anchored in a religion but shared by analogies of experience across cultural and religious backgrounds, not by identifying any 'lowest common denominator'.

Symbol A behaviour or artefact that both participates in and mediates the reality to which it points, usually by connotative means.

Techne Greek. Concerning technical aspects of creation or understanding.

Introduction

Background

Focus

Researching 'spirituality' is rather like researching 'inequality'; some distillation of focus is clearly necessary. Eventually, my somewhat loosely phrased brief to conduct some research into the spirituality of terminally ill people became a qualitative investigation of the 'sources of meaning and sense of self of people who are dying'. The absence of 'spirituality' or 'spiritual care' in the study title was a conscious decision. For some patients this type of vocabulary is charged with negative experiences of religion. This could have dissuaded their participation. I also wanted to disentangle the handling of existential questions from the exclusivities of religious practice. Patients were not to feel that they were disqualified from contributing because they did not attend a church or any other place of worship. Similarly, it was important not to foster any mistaken belief that, in some way, the study was connected with Spiritualism. Finally, the emphasis on personal meaning and identity reflects contemporary discussions of patients' spiritual needs and a general acceptance that while religious practice and spirituality may coincide, they are not necessarily synonymous (Brown and Williams 1993; Dyson and Cobb 1997). If this is so, the problem of recognizing how patients express their spiritual concerns when they do not use a religious vocabulary arises. The quest for a non-religious 'language of spirit' thus became an important focus, accompanied by a desire to explore what patients might use this language to say about themselves and their situation.

Terminology

Although 'spirituality' notoriously evades dictionary definitions, it sits fairly comfortably in the glossary. When the term arises in this book it refers to the interpretative story and ensuing values of an experience that is regarded as both human and ultimate. Spirituality is not necessarily anchored in a religion and it is not shared in the sense of a lowest common denominator, but by analogies of experience across cultural or religious boundaries. Ideally, but not necessarily, spiritual awareness and religious practice coincide. A religion is the life complex of practices, norms and structures of a community that find their origin in a founding spiritual revelation. Any religious development or articulation of spiritual experience is always a secondary process. Scant academic attention, however, has been paid to religion's primary import, which Dillistone (1955: 153) describes as supporting individuals in their 'steady advance to wholeness'. Most studies depict religious ritual and points of dogma or consider religious participation in terms of social cohesion. They contain frustratingly little reference to the human struggle for ultimate meaning and purpose. Given that spirituality discloses to us the 'really real' (Geertz 1973: 125) in that it provides the most fundamental and comprehensive account of life and its underlying value, however, it is about this struggle.

Nevertheless, as the following example shows, the combination of human and ultimate meaning that characterizes spiritually significant events or experiences is invariably easier to recognize than it is to explain. Hazel, frail and over eighty, refused to allow her nurses to clear some dead flowers from her bedside locker. This insistence was benignly viewed as a personal eccentricity until Hazel explained she was keeping the dead blooms because, as she watched the petals fall, 'They help me to let go. Although they have left this life, if you look carefully, you can see some are shooting up towards heaven; the ones with seedpods. Those seeds won't grow, of course, but the thought is heavenwards ... I do wonder what it's like after you're dead.'

Paradoxically, Hazel's flowers convey the comforting possibility of value and beauty, even in decay. By their own dying they also promise and withhold fertility and future life, keeping in creative tension the sense of threshold and wonder expressed in her final comment. Although not symbolic in any socially significant sense, the flowers draw attention to aspects of reality that generally tend to be overlooked and, by so doing, validate and comfort an elderly and isolated woman in ways that could easily have been dismissed by an overzealous urge to tidy.

This story, from a doctor who cared for a paralysed woman in rural France, carries similar implications. Although the woman was unable to speak, her nurses noticed she seemed to attach some significance to the Angelus ringing from a nearby church. When they arrived with her midday meal, she would indicate with her eyes for the window to be opened, to hear the bells more clearly. Blushing as she told me, her doctor felt that the combination of feeding and listening was more nourishing for her patient than either would have been alone, 'although I've no evidence for this. I mean, how could you show it?'

When listening to those who care for dying people speak about spirituality, I have always been struck by their need to resort to anecdotal material. Very often this need elicits an unease somewhat at odds with their otherwise positivist convictions. Many experienced people clearly feel constrained by the narrowness of prevailing notions of 'legitimate' or valid knowledge. Comments such as, 'I realize that this isn't scientific, but ...' or, 'I don't know how you measure this sort of thing, but this is what spiritual needs are all about' are far from uncommon. This tension first alerted me to the potential of story to disclose something new and relevant and the refusal of these disclosures to disappear because—not withstanding the pun, they do not count. Not all statements that are true correlate with what is 'out there in the world'. Stories are coherent statements of truth when they broadly make some sense of life—even if this sense resists easy encapsulation. As practitioners realize, a lack of empirical verifiability does not indicate a lack of meaning. Ignoring a good story is sometimes perilous to truth.

Another consultant, for instance, once spoke of a particularly withdrawn and silent patient. One Friday evening, when he was in a hurry to leave work, this man was sitting in the hospice foyer. Expecting little more than a quick acknowledgement, the consultant was surprised to find himself drawn into conversation. Forced to make his apologies, he explained that he was rushing to head off on a fishing trip. The man's eyes lit up. Fishing was his hobby. The following week he asked about the trip. As time passed, the consultant explained how he felt 'fishing talk' became a safe way of approaching threatening aspects of death and dying with this man. One day, the patient asked his wife to bring in his favourite rod. He and the consultant admired it in the garden where the man cast a perfect arc before returning to bed. He died peacefully only a few hours later. Somehow, his consultant felt, all of this carried a spiritual significance he could not quite put his finger on.

Criteria of appreciation

One of the aims of this book is to rehabilitate confidence in stories and experiences such as the ones described above as potential vehicles of spiritual meaning. I try to show how they can reveal an ultimately significant dimension in the here and now of daily life. In an era dominated by positivist enquiry this is not an entirely uncontroversial ambition. We tend to believe that there are two languages in which truth may be expressed: the language of numbers and the language of words. On the whole, the former carries authority (Steiner 1969: 31–56). What this book questions is not the undoubted achievements of empiricism but its monopolistic claims to knowledge. Spirituality resists tidy categorizations. Like the horizon, it continually retreats from our grasp. Patient's deepest 'sources of meaning', their most profound 'sense of self', do not fall within the arena of problem solving. The ordinary and the familiar mediate spiritual meaning certainly, but to be concerned with spirituality is also to be concerned with mystery. Problems are temporary stumbling blocks whereas mystery enfolds and draws one into itself: 'This is mystery meaning not unintelligibility but inexhaustible intelligibility' (Dunne 1975: 6). We, however, generally feel more comfortable with illusory boundaries. We think that unless a thing can be accurately classified and measured it is somehow less tangible, less real. In the circumstances addressed by this book, however, processes of interpretation are often more relevant than those of measurement and it is wiser to consider 'facts' in the same light as artefacts. Interestingly, facere originally meant to make something. Consequently, artistic integrity is a more appropriate concept for evaluating this book's truth claims than any technical 'objectivity'—a concept anyhow much questioned in contemporary philosophy. If the fundamental contribution of any recognizable theory is to explain 'the evidence at hand', qualitative and quantitative styles of research are, at least in this respect, comparable. For each, the good theory combines elements of invention with those of discovery and the role of communal discernment should not be neglected. 'Credibility' is thus another benchmark for this book. Its truth value and progressive force will be gauged by the degree to which its ideas evoke recognition, augment vision, cohere with wider debate and work on the ground.

Anyone searching these pages for a list of techniques or specific spiritual care practices, however, will be disappointed. Of course, this does not mean that nothing whatsoever 'useful' has emerged from listening to the experiences and thoughts of patients—far from it. Primarily, however, by giving a voice to terminally ill people, this book is something of a call to insecurity, to uncertainty and to recognizing the wisdom that lies in paradox. To 'ex plain' literally means to observe whatever emerges from a flattened landscape, whereas entering the terrain occupied by a dying person inevitably brings one face to face with complex situations and emotions. We live in a world where every movement is also a gesture and paradoxes such as loving and hating someone at the same time are commonplace. Rather than adopting an impossibly prescriptive tone, therefore, I hope this book will affect the kind of change that comes about when one is really 'taken up' by a poem, a painting or any work of art. As repressive regimes recognize only too effectively, good art exerts a normative truth claim. Good art is a positive and liberating moral force. For those who share the artist's vision, Hazel's wilting flowers are no longer simply rotting vegetation, but point to and present the wisdom and rhythms of nature. They suggest possibilities for a meaningful and apparently comforting transcendent order. This may sound somewhat portentous but 'transcendence' is only a matter of raising questions. It is simply an awareness of things that are outside one's everyday consciousness (Lonergan 1957: 636).

Perspective

We often glimpse or recognize in events a meaning we cannot describe, let alone explain. Life has always been larger than language. The expression of existential concerns, particularly if they carry metaphysical implications, is very much tied up with Polanyi's notion that we can know more than we can say (Torrance 1980). What, therefore, is the existential purchase of the stories I have cited? How far do they really take us? They may valuably be interpreted in psychological terms, but do they really tell us anything about the spiritual concerns of any patient? Palliative care prides itself as a multi-disciplinary field. To pursue these questions as far as I am able (which is certainly not to say they may be pursued no further), I have written this book from the perspective of pastoral theology. The research it describes complies with the highest standards of qualitative research, but it is also an example of theological anthropology.

Theology offers theory of ontological import (that is, relating to the nature or essence of being or existence) from the perspective of the ultimate concerns of its subject in relation to a range of features of reality such as life, death, happiness or goodness. Other disciplines handle these topics with tremendous insight, but theology searches for 'the meaning that gives meaning to all meanings' (Tillich 1962: 47). Sociology may study epidemiological and other aspects of mortality, psychology may ask, 'What is it like to die?' and 'What does my dying mean to me?', but neither discipline asks, 'Am I related to anything infinite or of ultimate meaning?' For many people facing death, however, it is hard to see how this question might seem less than relevant. The metaphysical search is necessarily an exercise in analogy because there is no specifically theological vocabulary. By definition, infinity or the ultimate eludes the formulations of finite, contingent creatures. Consequently, theologians can only try to show spirituality as it arises in real situations and by relying upon terminology borrowed from many sources. All disciplines, however, can only grasp the finite nature of beings in the context of some awareness of infinity, just as we may appreciate a frontier only because we have some implicit notion of the unlimited. A theological statement simply attempts to explain human experience at its deepest level and, like any other theory, must be judged by its ability to mediate and interpret its object.

Traditionally, theology handles spiritual awareness in terms of the experience and language of grace (Haight 1979). The graced experience is not of our own making but, like Hazel's appreciation of her flowers, may break unexpectedly into consciousness. Calling to mind James's (1902) and Hay's (1990) collected examples of unexpected 'spiritual experiences', Tillich (Boulad 1991: 149–50) emphasizes the gratuity of this offer: 'Grace strikes us when we walk through the dark valley of a meaningless and empty life ... It strikes when, year after year, the longed-for perfect life does not appear, when the old compulsions reign within us ... when despair destroys all hope and courage. Sometimes at that moment a wave of light breaks into our darkness, and it is as though a voice were saying, "You are accepted!" Nothing is demanded of this experience, no moral or intellectual presupposition, nothing but acceptance.'

At such a moment, despite any contradicting circumstances, one simply knows there is 'ground beneath one's feet'. Even one's finite existence may be experienced as a gift, both to be received and shared with others (Roy 1994). Grace always transforms for the better, raising a person to a new kind of existence. Liberation is thus its hallmark, even if concrete circumstances remain unchanged. Given that we can detect its effects, yet not explain its cause, the graced experience is thus as much a question as it is an answer. In further paradox, grace is not distinctly experienced as such, but comes to people only via the concrete circumstances of their lives and personality.

This leads to a further distinguishing feature of the theological perspective. Drawing on theories of matter and form, act and potency, Rahner (1966) argues that matter determines spirit by being what spirit informs and spirit informs matter, making it to be what it is. In the human person they are simultaneously united, mutually and reciprocally causative of each other, yet also radically different. Theology thus assumes an element of the transcendent in personhood. Although bound to sensible data and to the world, this element comes into contact with the absolute. Theologically speaking, 'the individual is of unconditional worth, because at the deepest level the personal self is at one with Absolute Reality' (Davis 1994: 151). Put simply, we are all 'worth' more than even our worst action might suggest.

This brief résumé of the theological perspective is not presented in any dogmatic sense and for some it may counter contemporary notions of researcher impartiality. It is, however, impossible to write from a position of complete neutrality, especially where existential matters are concerned. The book that is written from 'nowhere' does not exist in any discipline. Here, I have simply acknowledged that understanding is both personally and historically anchored. Indeed, it is hard to know how any researcher could ever find a neutral starting point. As Hay and Nye (1998: 82) write in their study of the spirituality of children, 'We need a horizon to "place ourselves within a situation".' Recalling earlier notions of artistic appreciation, my aim is to achieve some 'fusion' (Gadamer 1978: 68) between this book's argument and the understandings of those who read it. This is a conversational model of knowledge where wisdom does not equate with hitting some theoretical 'bed rock', but the ability to sustain dialogue in an ongoing process of discovery. The most successful outcome is shared understanding and mutual transformation. We feel that we have received something new and helpful for negotiating life and that somehow we have been enriched as people.

Structure

The book is divided into four parts. Part 1 provides a theoretical support for the spiritual interpretation of patients' words and deeds. Arguing that we live and die in story, metaphor and symbol are presented as the 'tools' of story making. They mediate our understanding of ourselves and of our place in the world and legitimately refer beyond the world of tangible 'facts' to disclose dimensions of life that cannot otherwise be 'said'. Psychology, spirituality and religion are presented as stories with conflicting limits and it is their understanding of symbolic potency that determines where this limit is set. Part 1 also describes how the many examples of patient narrative and behaviour were collected, analysed and interpreted.

Firmly grounded in patient experience, Part 2 presents a non-religious 'language of spirit'. It shows how patients make spiritually significant statements, even if they are not conscious of their full import. There are three major aspects to this language, none of which is a rigid category. These are its context (language is always about something), its literary form, where the use of archaic language and humour is explored and its symbolic form, the ways in which the past rings through present events, or certain motifs of spirit regularly emerge. How patients mobilize ritual and are affected by the deeper meaning and paradoxes of silence are also considered.

Carefully interpreted from a broad and varied literature, patients' voices claim Part 3 as the lion's share. If Part 2 describes a language of spirit, Part 3 shows what patients use this language to say about their situation and their spiritual needs. To enable a systematic handling of material, the simple model of a prism is presented. Every facet of this prism is constructed from one of nine metaphors. Each metaphor both describes and mediates patients' experiences and the metaphors influence one another. The first five metaphors are those of temporality, of marginality and liminality (a sense of threshold), of control and of letting go. The sixth facet of the prism, however, presents the hero as the first of three archetypal figures. The seventh and eighth facets respectively reveal the archetypal mother and stranger. The final facet considers the potential for human experience to evoke a 'surplus of meaning' that not only exceeds immediate appearances, but also our capacity to put it into words.

Part 4 does not give hard and fast rules for meeting patients' spiritual needs, but encourages readers to find the deepest meanings in their own encounters with patients, to reflect as much upon how they are with people as upon what they do. Spiritual care, like a good story, demands a response from the whole person, not simply the intellect and what it might mean to be 'whole' is also considered. Although spiritual care can be delivered by quite ordinary means, we can only hope to pave the way for experiences we are actually powerless to make happen. To this end, however, some modest suggestions are made for the creation of a free and friendly interpersonal space where carers can hopefully 'be the way' that spiritual care is given, without 'being in the way' (Nouwen 1998: 79).

Part 1

Understanding spirituality: how far can story go?

Chapter 1

How stories create and disclose meaning

Introduction

Spirituality may refuse to be pinned down in any definitive sense, but this does not mean it is impossible to recognize or discuss spiritual issues in ways that are cognitively valid. Indeed, some truths make their presence felt only because they continually withdraw from our grasp. To hear the spiritual needs of patients it is vital to appreciate the poetic function of language (which here includes all modes of communication, including body language). This is because language is sometimes most truthful when it enters into 'fiction', showing us truths that cannot be expressed literally or confirmed empirically.

Celina was a 38-year-old Ghanaian woman admitted to St Christopher's during an acute sickle cell crisis. Each crisis was more debilitating than the previous and her periods of remission were becoming shorter. Her admission coincided with my period of data collection and I was working as a nursing auxiliary/participant observer (see Chapter 3). Caring for Celina was challenging. She rang her bell frequently, making minor requests in an irritating, whining voice. Although seriously overweight and consequently hard to nurse, Celina ate only fattening food. She hated the night staff to leave her, but seemed to knowingly push their patience by constantly reciting her litany of misery. Celina's only family in the UK, her two children aged nine and seven, were in the care of the social services. Understandably, she wept, 'I am so far from my home and my people. No one here knows my ways. How can you as a white woman understand what it is like for me to be facing death? In Africa, everything to do with death is darkness. It is not the same for you here.' It was evening and sighing deeply, Celina indicated towards the night with a sweeping gesture. Illuminated only by a dim night-light, remnants of various packets of biscuits lay in her tangled sheets. Even during the day her curtains were closed and Celina slept in brief snatches, unable to tolerate the light, yet seemingly afraid of the dark. Although tense and agitated, she resisted any suggestions of evening sedation. Almost as a last resort I asked whether she would like to hear a story. She looked at me with some surprise: 'What story is this?' 'It is the story of a man in great danger whose deepest fear proves to be his friend.' 'Yes, I will listen to this story', and so, in the quiet side room, almost of its own volition—certainly without any forward planning on my part, the following tale unfolded. It exists in many forms, but the main themes (adapted here from Dass and Gormon 1985: 3–4) consist of an experienced diver swimming alone in deep water. Suddenly, he is doubled over with cramps so bad that he cannot even loosen his weight belt. His oxygen cylinder is nearly empty. As he sinks, his overwhelming sensation is one of panic. To make matter worse, he feels a prodding under his armpit. His terror intensifies. Sharks are a real possibility. Close to despair, the diver's whole being cries out for help. Then he realizes that his arm is actually being lifted. A moment later, he is looking into an eye that seems to be smiling. It is the eye of a dolphin. Flooded with relief, limp with exhaustion, the diver knows that he is saved. The dolphin brings him into waters so shallow he even wonders whether it might be beached, but the creature does not seem to want to leave him. The diver removes his equipment and returns naked to the water. The two play and splash together in the sunshine until, with a single sound, the dolphin swims out to sea, pausing only once to look back.

As she listened, Celina visibly relaxed. She closed her eyes, even smiled at the playful episode. Afterwards, a tear ran down her cheek: 'That is the most beautiful story I have ever heard—calming, beautiful. Thank you.' Albeit only for a short period, she gently drifted to sleep. Perhaps we should not be surprised by the story's capacity to traverse immense distances of culture and difference, or by its ability to comfort an anxious woman far from home. The universal character of myth or parable is well documented. As Celina's tear testifies, these are stories whose 'inner' meaning addresses one's entire being, not simply the intellect. Almost certainly, the intimations of mortality that imbibe the dolphin rescue with many of the qualities of a 'limit' situation—fear of the unknown, loss of control—would have been too frightening for Celina to hear in any other form. Dolphins, however, have long been associated with the extremes of human existence. Aboriginal accounts of creation describe the breath and bone lent to the first people by a dolphin. In Greek mythology they transport the dead to the underworld. These 'delphys', however, also invoke the transformational power of the womb, the literal meaning of their name, and the passage from death to rebirth.

Much as music liberates us from ordinary time, story also has a capacity to subvert conventional expectation. One's deepest fear can thus be revealed as a friend. Were this meaning expressed in balder more literal terms, however, it probably would not be accepted. Certainly, whenever such 'translations' are attempted, there is some loss of meaning, of subtlety, or the invitational quality of the story is violated. To translate once meant to betray, or as a rather beautiful Vietnamese saying puts it, 'to clips the bird's wings'. Story provokes us to enter its own world. Recruiting the reader or listener's imagination, it conjures into being that of which it speaks. The poetic function does not require external validation because it does not assert that something is true, it makes that truth real for us (Eliot 1933).

The 'storied' self

Story is more than just an occasional diversion: 'Poetically man dwells' (Heidegger 1976: 131). We live and die in story and there is no clear demarcation between literal and symbolic language. Every time we (re)describe our life's events, we are both providing and discovering underlying patterns of meaning. We are extracting a 'configuration' from what would otherwise be unrelated episodes and incidents, a mere 'succession' of events (Ricouer 1981: 278). The photographic montage where images of children, grandchildren, holidays, weddings and so forth are arranged into a meaningful whole is the visual equivalent. One patient described such a picture as, 'helping to draw life's strings together'. Sara, a young teacher, wrote the following poem. Her various hairstyles seem to be a 'configuring' motif.

> History of a head of hair
>
> At 12, long hair, "Big girl now", up
> to town—
> snip, snip, boo, hoo. Lots of, "You've
> had your hair cut." "I know."
> Never again—until aged 30
> crowning glory
> old men in pubs, some memory
> arose
> of a long lost love.
> They arose, approached, said
> "Never have it cut my dear." "No,
> OK."
> At 30, deep breath—
> Hack, hack. " … and this is the back."
> Flash in a mirror—all curls in a perm.
> Children were shocked, frightened.
> My voice from somebody else's body.
> One said, "You look like a bog brush."
> Many years later—to hospital,
> (shaved head for operation)
> then radiotherapy—came out in
> lumps and clumps.

> Bought a wig. "You look 16 again",
> said my mother.
> Now it's regrown, I feel like Tufty
> the squirrel
> but Adrian (Herr Doktor) keeps me
> looking human
> with the magic touch
> while Becci clips my claws.

Many women find losing their hair as great an assault to personal identity and self-esteem as their experience of a mastectomy (Freedman 1994). Legend, film and fable also betray the significance of hair: 'Rapunzel, Rapunzel, let down your golden hair'; 'Ryan's daughter' is shorn as punishment; Goldilocks is recognizable from her tresses; hairless Samson is doomed. Hair symbolizes power and life, perhaps explaining why some people suffering from psychosis or schizophrenia panic at the prospect of it being cut (Brun *et al.* 1993: 124) and why it makes sense for a terminally ill woman to reflect upon her life in terms of her various haircuts.

There is little doubt that our sense of who we are is sustained and mediated by narrative processes. The experience of serious illness may not shatter language in the ways described by Scarry's (1985) work on victims of acute torture, but it does have a tremendously undermining capacity. The harder it becomes for a sick person to 'inscribe' their various roles into the world, to predict the outcome of certain 'story lines' ('Will I finish my degree?' 'Will we go on holiday this year?' 'Will I see my son's next birthday?'), the greater seems the threat of self-dissolution. The 'career' of a terminally ill person also has a narrative structure (Charmaz 1983; Mathieson and Hendrikus 1995*a*). Catastrophic or puzzling incidents are 'retold' in ways that make them and the future bearable. We are all the 'readers' as well as the narrators of our life's events and our understanding of them is necessarily provisional. From the vantage point of middle age, one's twenties are seen in a very different light from that of one's youth. When listening to patients it is naïve to assume they are simply (re)describing experiences, or that their deepest beliefs are immediately accessible to consciousness. They may actually be searching, or fine honing their understanding, as they speak.

Narrative is often organized as a series of events—as with Sara's hairstyles—but sometimes this sequence, 'is only a net whereby to catch something else, the real theme may be, and perhaps usually is, something that has no sequence in it' (Lewis 1982: 17). Sara, for example, not only locates suffering, places and events in a meaningful order, but seems to open the future to some kind of positive ending, to a 'magic touch' (Adrian was her hairdresser). Stories can be quite unlike 'real life' in outward appearances, yet show us something about reality at a deeper level. They allow us to encounter mystery or to awaken a sense of otherness or possibility. The critical question, of course, is their degree of existential commitment. Does Sara's 'magic touch' simply suggest another better hairstyle or does it imply transformations of another order? Similarly, is it reasonable to wonder whether the dolphin rescue is somehow spiritually significant, whether it discloses a dimension of ultimate security in even the most precarious of human situations? Could its sharing qualify as an example of spiritual care?

Many will regard the rescue simply as a mildly sentimental anecdote. Those who examine stories in structural terms will detect mythologies of descent and resurrection, classically typified by Demeter and Persephone's journeys to and from the underworld, or more closely by Jonah and the whale. In apparently a disaster, the whale carries Jonah, the archetypal refusing man, safely to dry land. If the story is read psychologically, however, it could symbolize an encounter with repressed or subconscious material that is eventually successfully integrated. Theologically interpreted, both the story and its telling stand as examples of 'graced moments'. Each has a quality of gift, an unanticipated finding of somewhere—albeit temporarily—'safe to stand'. None of these competing interpretations, however, is exclusive or exhaustive and none necessarily 'disproves' any other. What is beyond dispute is that each vantage point depends on the same material: the lone swimmer, the dolphin and the vastness of the ocean. The story is powerful because it exploits the disclosive potential of these symbols and may be read metaphorically. Symbol and metaphor are two powerful story-making 'tools' and patients use them to draw attention to aspects of human experience that are generally overlooked. The crucial point, however, remains whether this experience is spiritually significant, whether it carries any ultimate meaning. In short, just how far can any story take us?

A problem of limit

The apparently simple question posed above has inspired a vast and complex philosophical literature whose close discussion unfortunately exceeds the parameters of this book. Nevertheless, to be concerned with how patients express their spirituality is to query whether language can have any real purchase over aspects of life that raise 'difficult' questions: 'Who am I?' 'Why must I suffer?' 'Why should anything, rather than nothing, exist?' 'What happens after death?' These are problems that challenge the limits of human understanding and in approaching them it is helpful to recognize that reality does not exist either in our heads or out in the world, but in how the two relate in language (Crossan 1975: 37). Trying to think without resorting to any kind of language is like asking how we might feel had we never been born.

Although we cannot transcend the medium of language, this does not mean that we are completely unable to reflect on the silent mysteries of our lives. Crossan (1975: 44) suggests that we imagine language as a raft. We may not speak empirically of the silent unknowing upon which our raft floats, but we can ponder the surrounding water. Ultimate meaning, he maintains, is disclosed where raft and water meet—at the point that is never 'only raft' or 'only water'. We can no more escape from language than we can sail directly into the wind, but our most exciting encounters take place when we sail as close as possible to the wind. The quest to recognize patients' spiritual concerns, to identify their sources of meaning and to understand their sense of self carries us to this limit. It will be seen that by mobilizing symbols and metaphor, patients' words and deeds can sail very close to the wind indeed.

Symbols and metaphor give us access to dimensions of meaning that lie beyond any literal telling. They show us what we cannot say and are able to mediate profound depths in quite ordinary events. Take, for example, the patient who described herself as 'spiritually comforted' because her nurse fetched her a cool pillowcase when she felt feverish. To understand the nurse's care in terms of a symbolic action is to recognize how 'the way care is given can reach the most hidden places' (Dame Cicely Saunders, in Kearney1996: 12). Similarly, to appreciate the disclosive potential of metaphor is to realize that patients do not need a specifically religious language to express their spiritual concerns and to construct the 'stories' that bring meaning to their lives. To avoid a narrow and superficial analysis of patient spirituality, therefore, some theoretical understanding of symbol and metaphor is vital.

Symbol and metaphor: the tools of story making

Symbol

It is important to understand that a symbol is not the same as a sign, signal or model (Fawcett 1970). A sign—EXIT or WC—denotes a specific object. It is the product of a common heritage and typifies objective thinking. A factory hooter is a signal. It may evoke certain feelings, but its disclosive potential is also limited. The same point applies to models, which can represent the exact knowledge of a thing (a scale train), or be analogical (collected cigarette ends denoting a smoker's lungs) (Soskice 1987: 101). A model is defined by its use as such and its reference is always limited in some way.

Clearly unable to provide descriptive models, anyone exploring spiritual issues is forced to rely upon the disclosive potential of symbols. Unlike models, symbols are not created but emerge spontaneously. The most powerful—earth, fire and water—are universal. Different symbols speak more loudly for different groups and cycles of disuse naturally occur. The symbol that is constantly repeated loses its creative power. To retain vitality it must be re-interpreted within fresh contexts. Human inclination is such, however, that this process easily degenerates into a fixed familiarity. In art, for instance, even the avant-garde will eventually fail to show the world in a new and refreshing light. Alternatively, a powerful symbol opens up what could not otherwise be apprehended. It suggests possibilities closed either to the signal or the sign. Derived from the Greek 'symballein', meaning 'to connect', a symbol is primarily connotative. It can embrace any facet of experience and hold together apparently contradictory features: the bush that burns but is not consumed, the 'wise fool' or 'silent music' (Johnston 1974). These paradoxical statements mark the limit of intellectual vision, but they are not nonsensical. We instinctively recognize their meaning.

The most distinguishing feature of a symbol is that it participates in the reality to which it points. Thus, a flame can symbolize hope and security because it warms and protects, but it also shares the destructive and purifying potential of anger, another of its symbolic meanings. In both cases, the flame actually mediates that which it symbolizes. This simple example not only shows how a symbol is directly untranslatable but also that its meaning is capable of indefinite growth as it evokes wide and varying associations, unlocking levels of reality which could not otherwise be apprehended. A symbol's point of reference can thus lie beyond the reach of empirical investigation (Tillich 1964a).

Symbols, however, do not assert a reality different to that assumed by the natural sciences. Understanding that reality has a dimension that cannot be described empirically and that meaning unfolds in the context of relationship; they are an expression of depth and inclusion (Frankl 1976: 189). Inviting us to a deeper understanding of reality, the symbol enables us to move from one layer of meaning to another. Its claims to knowledge, however, must be entered to be understood—and then only ever partially. A powerful symbol can also show us aspects of ourselves that we may consciously avoid and different symbols serve best at different stages in life. As any sensitive practitioner of palliative care knows, to impose ultimate categories on people engaged with penultimates is harmful. This is because symbols stimulate a deep response. They take hold of the individual— not vice versa, grasping their apprehending subject with an authenticity so profound that encounter replaces 'talk about' them. Innately powerful and expressive of the realities to which it points, a symbol can demand the highest responsive interpretation. As the poet W. B. Yeats recognized, 'He that sings a lasting song/Thinks in a marrow bone' (Smith 1987: 24). When the bush burned Moses removed his shoes and when we are touched deeply by a symbol we may experience an inner correlation with whatever it is that the symbol is mediating. Thus a 'peace garden' not only reveals something about the nature of peace, it can produce a sense of peacefulness in its visitors. This correlation makes it possible for Tillich (Hook 1962: 5) to write, 'Symbols of the Holy reveal something of the "Holy-Itself" and produce the experience of holiness in persons and groups.' To be holy is simply to experience oneself as whole. If only for a split second and regardless of external appearances, nothing needs to be added to, or removed from, one's situation to enhance this sense of completeness. Such moments may be rare, but they are recognizable. It is not inconceivable that Hazel valued her dying flowers or the French woman wanted to hear the Angelus ringing as she ate, because these were moments when they felt whole. Acting as a powerful medium that extends vision and stimulates imagination, a symbol—whether a ringing bell or a dying flower, can deepen human understanding so that even apparently unbearable situations may become tolerable. Given that the potency of any symbol may be judged only by its consequences, the grounds for this audacious claim lie only in the apparent satisfaction of both patients.

Symbol and meaning raise human life above the level of mere sensation and the most powerful symbol of all is the human person. The peace, justice or love mediated by individuals such as Gandhi, Martin Luther King or Mother Teresa transcend conventional expectations. Those who might object that a person can never be, 'only a symbol', might consider whether a person can be 'only' a 'fact literally recorded'. They are also well advised to recollect the absence of any sharp distinction between literal or historical 'facts' and their symbolic contextual meaning. Finally, the inaccessibility of a symbol to a direct translation means that the human person can never be completely known. There is always something more to learn. As Crossan's raft reminds us, life is larger than language. Through metaphor, however, we can articulate the 'silent side' of many frontiers.

Metaphor

It is impossible to appreciate certain depths of meaning in patient narrative without understanding the disclosive potential and working of metaphor. When we are, 'speaking about one thing in terms which are seen to be suggestive of another', we are using metaphor (Soskice 1987: 15). The functioning of metaphor, however, is somewhat mysterious. It is more easily approached in terms of negatives: metaphor does not simply decorate 'proper' speech. There are not two meanings for every metaphor—one literal and one metaphoric, so that a metaphor is both true and false at the same time. Metaphoric truth is not inferior to literal truth because it is philosophically impossible to distinguish literal from metaphoric language. It is thus a false assumption that to carry any cognitive weight, a metaphor must always be reducible to a literal statement (Soskice 1987: 68).

The economy with which a good metaphor conveys complex thoughts and feelings is impressive. I was very struck by a patient who described himself as living, 'on microwave time'. In microwave cookery, the last few minutes, when a dish is left to stand, are the most crucial. This patient had recently completed a course of chemotherapy and I wondered whether, obliquely or even subconsciously, he was speaking of his own waiting for an outcome. Perhaps he was acknowledging that, despite his outward passivity, his 'inner world' was still highly active and in ways that mattered.

A good metaphor invites interpretations from many angles. There is never an exact literal equivalent. Furthermore, one does not have to listen to many patients, 'swimming for the shore', 'being hit by a sledgehammer' or 'riding a roller coaster' to realize they are not speaking with any sense of these metaphors being inferior to literal language or with any intention to deceive—an accusation often made against metaphor. Neither is there any sense of them 'translating' a previously conceived 'literal' meaning. Like the images patients produce during art therapy (Connell 1998), metaphor gives them a way of expressing thoughts and feelings that can perhaps be said in no other way. Importantly, when an effective metaphor makes an 'impossible utterance', its meaning is often easily recognized. We wonder why we could not 'see' before what now seems so obvious.

Aristotle writes in his Poetics that the greatest thing for a person to be is a 'master of metaphor' since it is an ability that, despite being present from quite early childhood, cannot be learnt from others. Metaphor, he continues, is a sign of genius because it implies an intuitive sense of similarity in 'dissimilars'. Certainly, the effective metaphor embodies a tension between 'what is' and 'what is not'. For the man mentioned above, something about his experience of terminal illness resonated with his observations of microwave cooking—although microwave cuisine is definitely not about dying. It is the tension between the two states of affairs—the 'is' and the 'is not'—that permits the novel and somewhat startling insights into his situation. By drawing our thinking in unanticipated directions metaphor shows us reality afresh.

The social context and relational networks that surround the creation of any metaphor ought not to be ignored. Without appreciating that the man 'on microwave time' was terminally ill, for instance, the potency of his utterance is reduced. 'Microwave time' may be a linguistic phenomenon, but it involves many associations, including the beliefs and intentions of both its speaker and its listener. Through such interacting networks, Soskice (1987) argues, metaphor realizes its creative potential. Any reduction to a literal paraphrase, attempted translation or 'peeling apart' of metaphoric and literal meaning is misguided and will incur some overall loss of meaning—or perhaps result in no meaning at all. The 'dictionary of metaphors' does not exist because the meaning of a metaphor does not lie at the level of specific words or linguistic constructions— just as the meaning of a novel or a poem does not lie in the sum of its sentences.

Nevertheless, a powerful metaphor will address us at a deep and personal level and in ways closer to processes of encounter than of translation. Perhaps this risk of encounter explains why patients' 'throwaway' lines are sometimes glossed over or ignored by carers. As, for example, by the nurse who, without even a sympathetic smile, simply continued to dress her patient's heels while he explained they were sore because he was 'kicking the bucket for too long'. Alas, it is harder for patients to immure themselves from the effects of metaphor and Sontag (1978) eloquently describes how metaphors of contagion, warfare and contamination influence the experiences and actions of cancer patients. The 'total liberation' from metaphor to which she aspires, however, is impossible. The best she can hope for is to replace repressive or hurtful metaphors with kindlier sets of associations. This is because all dimensions of human life, even those we consider to be most 'objectively real', are interpreted and mediated by metaphor.

We may generally be unaware of our thoughts and perceptions being mediated by systematic and coherent networks of metaphoric associations, but Lakoff and Johnson (1980) argue that metaphor is as essential to our understanding of the world as is our sense of touch. Our capacity for metaphor is actually physically grounded—we associate alert with up, passive with down. Similarly, childhood experiences of containment, conditioned by the varying responses of family members, develop our 'inside–outside' orientations. How we talk about, conceive of and experience life are all metaphorically structured. We live by metaphor. For example, when we describe a dispute in terms of 'demolishing' the opposition, 'defending' a point of view or making 'indefensible' claims, each statement is rooted in the metaphor 'argument is war'. We actually see the person we are arguing with as an opponent and know that we will either win or lose. 'Argument is war' is a metaphor by which Western culture lives. It powerfully mediates our experience of reality. Inevitably, cultural variations in metaphor produce other understandings. Bharati (1985), for example, discusses the role of culture in the formation of the penetrable boundaries of the Hindu body-self.

Metaphor can transcend dictates of logic and reason. Seeing the 'like' in the 'unlike' allows the laws of sympathetic magic to operate in everyday life (Rozin *et al.* 1986) so that, under the law of contagion, clothes worn by a disliked person are regarded as soiled even after washing. Under the law of similarity, people will not eat faecal-shaped chocolate or are less accurate throwing darts at a picture of a friend than an enemy. Interestingly, many patients admitted to St Christopher's for 'respite care' do not return home but die in the hospice. Such patients are clearly extremely ill on admission and one experienced consultant laughingly remarked that although their referring practitioners realized this, she felt they disliked booking admissions for 'terminal care' because 'They're scared of hexing them; if they say it, or write it down, it might happen!'

The argument that metaphors mediate, influence and disclose our reality for us, repudiates notions of pure objectivity or pure subjectivity. This does not equate with being anti formal scientific theory. Rather, the scientific model ought to be regarded as a consistent set of metaphors that applies only in restricted situations. It is quite another thing, to conclude it is an accurate or literal reflection of all reality. The creative aspect of metaphor does not oppose processes of scientific explanation, however, because it is central to their working. Billiard balls allow the properties of gases to be discussed, light is presented in terms of particles or rays and genetic material as Morse code and the enigmas of space are handled in terms of 'black holes'. Physiologists speak in terms of oxygen 'debts' and ecologists of 'hierarchies' and 'niches'. Because a metaphor is not a strict definition, it allows for constant revisions of meaning. Consequently, science tends to rely more heavily upon metaphor when it does not fully comprehend a situation. In this respect, it is hard to distinguish from many discussions of human spirituality. There is often little difference in the referential value of a religious and a scientific metaphor. The 'good shepherd', for instance, is as referentially legitimate as the 'laws of nature'. Nevertheless, there is a common assumption that scientists resort to metaphor only to make complex theories available to non-scientists. This is not the case. Scientists exploit metaphor as much as theologians because it also allows them, at least partially, to depict reality without needing to be irreducibly definitive. They too can refer without needing to define; they too can speak before they fully understand what it is they are talking about. By combining the two processes of invention—discovery and creation—metaphor names that which previously had no name and this applies as much in the natural sciences as in discussions of human spirituality. The critical factor for both parties is whether a metaphor 'works on the ground'. Is it helpful to think of 'junctions' as existing along nerves? Does the notion of ultimate meaning tally with aspects of human experience? This is the kind of critical reasoning by which all knowledge proceeds.

Metaphor and symbol operate where our prevailing sense of reality, Crossan's raft of language, meets the vast ocean of our unknowing. In ways that are cognitively acceptable, they both mediate and disclose to us hitherto unknown dimensions of our reality. They are 'tools' for 'touching' life at its deepest level so that Thich Nhat Hanh, a Vietnamese Buddhist Monk (Hanh 1993: preface) can write

> If you touch deeply the historical dimension,
>
> You find yourself in the Ultimate dimension.
>
> If you touch the Ultimate dimension,
>
> You have not left the historical dimension.

Spirituality is not an 'extra'ordinary feature of life but a suffusing dimension, mediated and disclosed to us by the workings of metaphor and symbol. Often, we simply fail to perceive its presence. Of course, it can be argued that the notion of ultimate meaning is at best misleading, at worst damaging and that psychology, not theology, reaches the furthest horizon of human meaning. In a climate where resources are tightly allocated, the co-standing of psychological and spiritual readings of human experience will undoubtedly influence future patterns of palliative care. There are signs, Hardy's (1987) title—*A psychology with a soul*, for instance, that the tenancy of spirituality within certain branches of psychology is fast becoming regarded as secure. While there are many areas of overlap, the critical difference between the two 'stories' lies in their interpretation of symbolic potency. This is not an issue tangential to spiritual needs but forces us to consider whether patients' words and deeds are always afforded their full dignity of meaning.

Chapter 2

Spirituality and psychology: stories with differing limits

Introduction

Although all Primary Care Trusts in the UK are encouraged to meet the spiritual needs of terminally ill people (Shipman *et al.* 2002) and despite a widespread recognition that health requires the presence of mental, physical and emotional well-being, not simply the absence of disease or infirmity (World Health Organization 1990), many professionals confess a lack of confidence in recognizing and responding to spiritual needs. This insecurity is perhaps demonstrated and, to some degree, counterbalanced by a tendency to think that if only we could identify discrete indicators of spiritual distress in a manner similar to that employed by many scales of psychological assessment, we could respond appropriately and so improve the lot of patients.

I wish to suggest that attempts to distinguish the spiritual from other aspects of human experience indicate a conceptual bondage more symptomatic of ways of talking, than of human modes of being. It is because spirituality evades both literal description and quantifiable analysis that we are forced to rely upon the disclosures of metaphor and symbol to expand our understanding of spiritual issues. Instinctively, we turn to poetry and the arts for a depth reading of reality. Shakespeare's *Hamlet* survives because successive generations recognize the authenticity of its truth claims. Unless we also learn to approach spirituality with subtlety and imagination there is a danger that taboo and insecurity will result in the denial of fundamental aspects of human experience, simply because they are not easily categorized. Many of the patients in this book address issues that arise at the frontier of existential understanding: the compatibility of justice and mercy, the purpose of human life—my life, the meaning of suffering or as one woman put it, 'Where is God in all this?'. Such problematics extend beyond the reach of the humanities, psychology, even of philosophy and it is not easy to listen to such struggling. One cannot help but wonder whether the inclination to compartmentalize spiritual issues highlights a tendency to intellectualize situations that ultimately require a response from us as whole people.

It is possible, however, to argue for a horizon of meaning that accommodates and relativizes all other interpretations of human life—even the empirically based. This furthest point resists total seizure, but it is incumbent upon us to find as many ways as possible of talking about the indefinable. The further into 'uncharted territories' we can honestly place our own existential 'stake', the more we give patients tacit permission to raise what they may otherwise feel are 'illegitimate' topics and the less likely we are to 'psychologize' spiritual issues by allowing our enquiries to fall short of any ultimate horizon of meaning. This tendency is surely recognized by patients who frequently preface their most profound and intimate disclosures with disclaimers such as 'I know you'll think I'm mad, but …'. By failing to recognize the potential depth of meaning contained in ordinary events we show that we have foreshortened our horizons of interpretation. We are selling patients' experiences short and may miss opportunities for fostering hope and comfort. Worse yet, we may approach patients with a reductive attitude, interpreting their intimations of spiritual awareness as signs of regression, denial, manifestations of an externalized father figure and so forth. These explanations, of course, may come into play, but they ought not to be reached for simply as a matter of course. Rather than judge the validity of another's experiences, we may be required to accept that a patient is in touch with something we may find inaccessible. Paradoxically, however, it is sometimes by acknowledging our own entry to unfamiliar areas that we can create an inviting space for others to enter.

Spirituality: a further look

When so many churches find it necessary to urge their visitors to adopt a respectful attitude, it hardly seems necessary to repeat that spiritual awareness and religion are not necessarily synonymous. Presumably the notice, 'this building is not a museum' outside Cologne cathedral is necessary, because to most people, this is exactly what the cathedral is (Hay 1987: 43). Anthropological accounts of spirituality draw attention to the human search for meaning and purpose. Frankl's (1992: preface) famous endorsement of Nietzsche's aphorism 'He who has a *why* to live can bear almost any *how*', has acquired almost shibboleth status for discussions of spirituality in palliative care. Numerous psychological studies, however, suggest that it is a mistake to limit human spirituality to a purely conceptual search. The heightened awareness of sportsmen, the 'inner time' and corporate mutuality shared by musicians and reports from individuals who feel they have transcended the boundaries of their everyday self, all point to a 'natural spirituality' in human beings that is partially characterized by an experiential element (Neitz and Spickard 1990). Even in the contemporary UK, between half and two-thirds of the population claim to have experienced a 'spiritually significant' event. The resultant feelings of awe, wonder and unity cause Hay (1990) who has documented these accounts, to root spiritual awareness in genetic predisposition, positively associating it with health and personal integration. Although writing as an empiricist, he endorses Rahner's theological argument that, even if all religions were one day to disappear, 'the transcendentally inherent in human life is such that [we] would still reach out towards that mystery which lies outside our control' (Rahner 1974: 160).

There are, however, arguments against aligning spiritual awareness exclusively with the extraordinary 'encounter', as much as there are reasons against confining it to a conceptual search for meaning. Spirituality is also potentially manifested in a number of generally accessible ordinary human activities. These serve as what Berger (1969) calls 'signals of transcendence'. He describes a mother soothing a frightened child late at night. By so doing, she intimates a belief in an ultimate reality or cosmic order, a trust in 'being', a conviction that 'all will be well'. If reality is co-extensive with natural reality she is serving the child an illusion, for all is clearly not well in the world. Yet, as Berger asks 'Is the mother lying?' Joyful play will similarly suspend general assumptions. In a step from chronos to kairos, from the measured time of the clock to a sense of timelessness, the adult is momentarily re-integrated with the infinity and deathlessness of childhood—where infinity means not an endless 'now' but being 'out of time'. It is plausible to regard any dislocation of conventional temporality as a sign of nascent spiritual awareness—an argument that will be developed later in the context of patients' varying perceptions of time.

Sequential models of personal development implicitly reserve spirituality for adulthood (Fowler 1981). Studies of childhood spirituality, however, also draw attention to ordinary activities (Hoffman 1992). Sometimes spirituality is described in terms of an 'inner life' in relation to physical reality, but to apply this understanding to children ignores discussions of emerging consciousness, the development of memory, attention span and categorizations of time. Furthermore, contemporary philosophy has virtually demolished the Cartesian position of an inner 'soul' acquiring all its information by reflecting upon itself (Kerr 1986). Hay and Nye (1998), therefore, identify four subcategories of childhood spirituality beginning with the experience of being in the *here and now*. Religious interest in this 'point mode' of concentration (Donaldson 1992) exists in many cultures, but they argue de Caussade's (1981) advocacy of the 'sacrament of the present moment' is most familiar in Western Christianity. Hay and Nye also mobilize the psychological concept of *tuning* to show how an intense experience such as bullying can prompt a spiritual crisis in a child, whereas their birthday party can induce powerful feelings of unity and belonging. An otherwise unremarkable activity such as learning to ride a new bike may constitute an experience of *flow* similar to the reports of skiers, rock climbers or chess players who interpret their experiences as spiritually significant. A final sub-category concerns *focusing*. Much discussed in the context of meditation, focusing carries implications of a kinaesthetic awareness, supporting the argument that embodied awareness is the natural knowing of young children. The four psychological categories, however, are not necessarily confined to childhood experience. When considering spirituality, to stress the cognitive dimension of personhood at the expense of the affective, social or physical, counters the holistic principles of palliative care and excludes the experiences of many people—especially those of children and of adults with learning difficulties (Vanier 1993).

Through the ages, various patterns of monastic formation and practices such as yoga and meditation have demonstrated how our spiritual and physical natures are not two Platonic 'inner' and 'outer' selves, but interpenetrating and mutually constitutive dimensions of the one human person. A useful analogy exists in the ancient Roman concept of the 'architectonic'. The 'architectonic' is that quality which pervades a structure with poise and beauty. It is no 'thing', yet neither is it 'nothing'. Dismantling a building or statue in its pursuit, however, will yield only rubble. Like spirituality, it is a distinctive, but not a distinct aspect of reality. This book's jettisoning of compartmentalized readings of human spirituality in favour of a dimensional approach merits one final point. Height, depth and breadth each have their own language, but to speak in terms of one does not mean the other two are ignored. Their presence is necessarily implicit. To speak of height, for example, without any conception of depth or breadth is meaningless. Similarly, spirituality is tacit in any discussion of patient experience, whether by doctors, social workers, providers of pastoral care or psychologists. Truth is not always the whole truth.

'Con-fusions'

Metaphysical terms sit uneasily in positivist mainstream psychology, but where people once approached religion for spiritual guidance, today they are more likely to turn for help to a psychotherapist, psychologist or counsellor. For many in search of integrity and inner healing, the traditional role of the priest has been usurped. Countless schools of psychotherapy claim to foster personal spiritual development. Nearly all, however, owe some debt to the writings of Carl Jung who famously observed that 'Among my patients in the second half of life—that is to say over 35—there has not been one whose problem in the last resort was not that of finding a religious outlook on life. It is safe to say that everyone of them fell ill because he had lost that which the living religions of every age had given to their followers, and none of them has really been healed who did not regain this religious outlook' (1961: 24).

Jung, however, claimed status only as an empiricist, recognizing that an affirmation of the psychic reality of ultimate reality neither affirms nor denies its ontological existence. Nevertheless, there is little doubt that his emphasis on the individual's drive or call to full humanity, his stress on inner exploration and personal experience and his reinstatement of the symbol as a valid form of knowing—all couched in a non-prescriptive respect for personhood—can sound seductively like a spiritual reading of the human situation. In one sense, this is hardly surprising. Methods and standpoints may differ, but spiritual and psychological explorations are both concerned with the same creature. Theology can no more exclude from 'soul' what conventionally belongs to 'psyche' than psychology can exclude from 'psyche' what traditionally is ascribed to the 'soul'. Similarly, neither discipline is inseparable from anthropology: the idea of man, his nature, mode of existence and destiny. A psychology founded exclusively on a scientific model, however, will always be frustrated by its inability to handle deeply personal questions regarding what we believe about the nature of human beings and our relationships. The originality of Jung's thinking, the pedestrian status of much of his terminology (extrovert, introvert, neurotic, complex and so on), and his major influence on contemporary psychotherapeutic practice, have a gone long way to broadening this restricted perspective, tempting some to regard his as a narrative that deals with ultimate issues. Nevertheless, as Jung freely acknowledged, in such matters he halts exactly where we would like to know more.

It is Jung's understanding of symbol that most distinguishes his reading of the human situation from a spiritual interpretation. Whilst it is relatively easy to account for the death of a symbol, it is altogether harder to explain its origin—not only in the sense of how it arises, but in terms of identifying its source of potency. Psychological explanations take one a long way with the first problem, but the latter is somewhat mysterious. From a spiritual perspective, life has a meaning that extends beyond, yet incorporates, the horizons of psychology. Expressed theologically, the action of Grace is a fundamental 'given' of human experience. Its origin lies outside human fabrication yet is expressed in the symbols and vocabulary of 'love', 'personhood' and 'creation'. Jung, however, regards symbols as powerful products of either the individual subconscious or of the collective unconscious. This has resulted in a 'constant confusing of collective (and "archetypal") with transpersonal and mystical ...

the tendency then is to take anything collective and call it spiritual, mystical, transpersonal' (Wilber 1996: 216).

Archetypes considered

Wilber is both timely and acute in drawing attention to Jung's concept of the archetype for it easily facilitates a certain 'fudging' of spiritual and psychological parameters of significance. Furthermore, although necessarily brief, this theoretical consideration will usefully anticipate and adumbrate later chapters concerning three archetypal mediators of patient experience. The archetypes or archetypal symbols are certain patterns and motifs that repeatedly occur in the mythology, tales and religious images of all people. For Jung, their origins lie deep in the collective unconscious of all mankind. At the same time, archetypes are innate predispositions occurring in the psyche of each individual. They are inferred from particular sets of circumstances or sensory impressions but are not apprehended directly. Two individuals, therefore, need not experience identical dreams for each dream to infer the same archetype. An archetype can be prompted (in Jungian terms 'constellated') by changes in the outer circumstances of an individual's life, on to which it will then be projected. Sometimes this leads to unexpected and highly charged emotions and behaviour whose consequences will vary, for the archetypes carry both a negative and a positive potential. So far, both theory and observation concur with existing reflections in palliative care (Bolen 1996; Kearney 2000; Wheelwright 1981). An important question, however, inevitably arises: do archetypes carry ultimate meaning, or is their import entirely psychological? Patients presented in Part 3 of this book suggest that the readings of depth psychology, valuable as they are, do not carry enquiry far enough. Experience thus intimates that what is true of psyche may be true of spirit, but not completely so.

Where Jung does turn to Ultimate issues, he does so in anthropomorphic fashion, speaking of the 'good' and 'bad' sides of God. His writing on 'integrating', 'becoming conscious of' or 'accepting' (all highly ambiguous terms) evil, fails to recognize that goodness and completeness are philosophically synonymous. Personal integration cannot be the addition of evil to good. Negativity is transformed because its privations are supplied. The privation of integrity cannot be integrated and this knowledge forces a choice between good and evil propounded by all spiritual traditions, so distinguishing those who have experienced the reality of the archetypes from believers (White 1960). Jung may also be criticized for not distinguishing the archetype of deity from symbols of the self and for failing to recognize that there is no convenient God against which to measure the image, as there is a natural mother or father. His view of all psychic happenings as real or 'psychic facts' inevitably gives rise to the (unanswered) question, what is a psychic 'falsehood'? The 'I Believe' of a credal proclamation may qualify as a psychic fact, but it also illustrates Jung's fundamental confusion of psychic fact and Truth. For the believer, dogmas make metaphorical and literal statements, not only about our selves, but about ultimate realities or Truth. Assent to propositions such as 'This is my Beloved Son' or 'There is only one God and Mohammed is his prophet' also require the exercise of judgement—a faculty somewhat neglected in Jungian thought. Finally, Jung regards dogma not only as a conscious response to and reflection upon experience, but as its substitute, protecting an ego too weak to cope with the forces of the unconscious. Many would respond that mature faith—the confidence that, perhaps in spite of appearances, life can be trusted—ought not to be so confidently equated with products of the unconscious. Such faith never damages but fulfils. It enlarges the archetypal experience in ways that undermine its claims to primacy. A Jungian analysis may awaken spiritual interest, but nowhere are the disclosure of ultimate meaning, life's potential for metaphysical encounter or the movement and experience of grace accepted in any cognitive sense. As Jung acceded, however, the legitimate concern of psychology is the phenomenon of spiritual experience as an activity of the psyche and its inner processes.

Nevertheless, despite the divergences briefly sketched here, Skynner (1976) argues that it is easy to see why spiritual discomfort should be regarded as entirely synonymous with psychological pain. In both cases, man's perception is distorted. Spiritual traditions speak of Samsara or the world of appearances. Psychotherapies speak of projection, withdrawal into fantasy or denial. From both perspectives, the individual is regarded as fragmented with personal blindness contributing to their suffering. Self-knowledge is the avenue to personal integrity and when disowned aspects of the personality become conscious, the 'lost sheep' is found, 'the prodigal' has returned. This can be a painful journey and both psychotherapy and sacred tradition require the searcher to stay in regular contact with a guide, guru, spiritual director or analyst. Having been through a similar experience, it is assumed that they will have a high degree of personal insight and sensitivity to the needs of others.

Psychotherapies aim for improved relationships, a secure identity, self-acceptance, openness and honesty. These are all attainable without requiring any exploration of life's deeper meaning and Skynner maintains that patients whose needs are entirely psychological can be distinguished from those who are 'more troubled about and interested in the meaning of their existence as a whole rather than the meaning of what happened to them yesterday or in their childhood or in the hopes and fears of what will happen to them tomorrow'

(Skynner 1976: 210). These words bear comparison with Kearney's description of spiritual pain, 'my experience is that with time it becomes possible to "sense", to "know" when the discomfort or pain has a spiritual origin. After meeting an individual in spiritual pain I find that terms like "suffering", "anguish" or "deep restlessness" most aptly describe the experience' (Kearney 1990: 50). As Kearney acknowledges, such intuitions are best supported in the cross-examining environment of a multi-disciplinary team.

The notion of an ordered intelligent universe tends to be central to most spiritual readings of the human condition, along with the conviction that immediate reality is permeated with deeper meaning. Prayer, meditation and mindfulness can foster perception of this meaning, so that, in Skynner's words (Skynner 1976: 214), 'a more subtle intelligence becomes available and begins to change the whole meaning and purpose of ordinary life'. Clearly, speculation of this nature is not part of any psychology, be it 'scientific' or 'humanist'. A search for a spiritual dimension that begins with disillusionment with one's ordinary self departs from the exact point psychological therapies generally seek to affirm and improve. Psychotherapy is about helping people to cope with daily life—such as earning a living or maintaining relationships, or at particularly times of stress, such as at divorce or bereavement. Spirituality may find expression in such moments but, for many, it is also concerned with our sense of connection to any 'cosmic design' or 'essential' that precedes our condition (Eliade 1957). From a spiritual perspective, what matters is how time and eternity converge and relate within each individual. Social and psychological variations in the experience of temporality are well documented. The critical issue, however, remains whether time has a symbolic dimension whose spiritual reading is ever warranted. For some this is a fanciful and misleading notion. Nevertheless, there are patients for whom, with advancing illness, time can become a far more mysterious and relative affair than was previously assumed.

Although constraints of space necessarily limit and simplify this handling of spiritual and psychological 'stories', certain differences in their existential purchase and remit do emerge. Divorced even from these brief considerations, the following accounts of data collection and interpretation would be severely denuded. As any skilled storyteller knows, preparing the ground is as important as the telling.

Chapter 3

Stories in the 'listening': collecting data

Participant observation

For this study I conducted a 5-week observational period on one of the hospice wards. Participant observation entails the systematic description of events, behaviours and artefacts. Immersing the researcher in the area of study, it assumes that observed behaviour sometimes indicates deeper values and beliefs. Observation ranges from the extremely focused to a more diffuse awareness (Marshall and Rossman 1989). Whilst also working as an auxiliary nurse I discretely recorded incidents and impressions on a secretarial dictaphone. I later wrote these up in a fieldwork journal.

Accommodating 17 patients, men and women in single-sex bays, the ward was laid out rather traditionally with four four-bedded bays off a main corridor. At the far end were two single side rooms and a small sitting room. Beside each bed stood a locker, easy chair and bedside table. Patients could bring anything from home that might reasonably be accommodated. One patient, Camilla, transformed her side room with her music centre, pictures, rugs and even her pet cat. Typically, however, beds were covered with attractive pale peach and green covers, co-ordinating well with the matching decor. Nevertheless, in comparison with more modern hospices, there was still the feel of a medical ward. On the opposite side of the corridor lay a number of bathrooms, a sluice, a smaller sitting room and the nurses' office. Large windows at the end of the corridor overlooked the well-tended garden, while the windows of the patient's bays gave to the smaller front garden and tennis courts opposite the hospice. All surrounded by mature tall trees, this created a pleasant outlook.

Staffing levels at St Christopher's are higher than in the National Health Service, something frequently remarked upon by patients and visitors. Other than auxiliary nurses, who have their own in-house training programme, all members of staff are qualified and there is no internal rotation of students. This undoubtedly fosters a sense of stability; staff know one another and they know what they are doing. Nurses wear a navy skirt, culottes or trousers with a grey polo shirt or pale blue blouse. The style is smart but casual and there is no distinction between the nursing ranks in terms of uniform, although name badges clearly state designation. My own badge was labelled 'researcher' although I wore a nurse's uniform. Every patient admitted to the ward received a leaflet from their welcoming nurse that outlined the nature of the research and my dual role. The leaflet also explained how my observations would not be concentrated on any particular patient. Even so, if anyone felt uneasy about the presence of a researcher on the ward they were urged to request that I not be involved in their care. In no way, it was emphasized, would this decision influence the standard of care they would receive. In the event, however, nobody did express feelings of disquiet.

Most days on the ward followed a familiar pattern: the morning shift for nurses commences at 07:30 hours and ends at 15:15 hours. Afternoons commence at 13:00 hours and end at 21:15 hours, while the night shift extends from 20:45 hours until 07:45 hours. Nursing care is organized in three teams and although I was observing all patients, I worked within one particular team. Each patient has their named nurse as a primary care giver who also acts as the liaison person for other members of staff. All shifts begin with a detailed description of each patient's condition over the previous 8 hours. The attention to detail at each 'hand over' is staggering with consideration extending to the needs of family and friends. Although care was never forced upon patients if they felt too ill, and they were free to request assistance at a time of day when they were feeling strongest, mornings were largely seen as the time for 'heavy' work: bathing, attending to bowel care, changing dressings. In the afternoon there was more time to sit with patients, although qualified nurses often seemed under pressure to write monstrously comprehensive care plans. Afternoons were also used for 'day-after-death' meetings where the recently bereaved would return to the ward to collect the death certificate, discuss the care of their relative and perhaps be taken to the mortuary chapel to view their body. Understandably, there was no predicting the length of time relatives might need. The atmosphere of the ward was generally calm and peaceful but all staff were engaged in a purposeful inter-weaving of activity.

St Christopher's advocates a multi-disciplinary model of care. Doctors, nurses, physiotherapists, chaplains, social workers and others discuss patients at a weekly ward meeting. Close attention is paid to the minutiae of each person's condition and home or family circumstances. Points of stress or pressure are identified and possible solutions discussed. My nursing background and previous experience of working with disabled people and their families undeniably provided a privileged point of access to the phenomena I wished to study. Nevertheless, it was still necessary to 'earn' the confidence of staff on the ward and most of my energies were initially spent informally explaining what the study was about and establishing myself as someone to whom patients could be entrusted. In the early days, I occasionally felt that nurses were hovering to observe how I interacted with patients, whether they felt at ease with me.

On my first morning on the ward, prayers were said at the end of the bays. Apparently this was a departure from convention and I felt it was performed for my benefit. Clearly, there was a need to reassure staff that I was not 'checking up' on any aspect of practice. The title of the study ('Sources of meaning and sense of self in people who are dying') was helpful here and I never observed prayers being formally said again. Perhaps my presence did initially distort the dynamics between staff, or staff and patients, but as time went by I began to feel confident that my observational role had been comfortably accommodated and that it felt natural to have me around.

I had requested to work as an auxiliary rather than a staff nurse as I felt that this would release me from responsibilities that may have caused tensions between the role of participant observer and of carer. I also felt that it would help to maintain my identity as nurse, but 'other', amongst staff. Auxiliary nurses would be aware that I was not fully 'one of them', while staff nurses would be aware that I was not to be regarded as their professional equal.

Only once was this ambiguous status directly challenged when, over the supper break one evening, I was asked by the nurse in charge whether I would look after the drug keys while she left the ward. The keys are an instantly recognizable symbol of authority and responsibility for all nurses and I would have been the only qualified member of staff on duty. Their acceptance felt ethically and methodologically inappropriate: in the event of an emergency I do not possess specialist training in palliative care and the safety of patients was potentially threatened. Secondly, it felt like too radical a departure from my role of observer. I was supernumerary to staffing levels and it was important to periodically remind staff of this fact if I was to avoid the dangers of entering totally into the role of nurse and jeopardizing my role as researcher. There was a fine balance to be struck between struggling to gain acceptance, yet preserving that distinguishing element of the 'stranger' about myself (Simmel 1950).

It was clearly impossible, however, to operate as a *tabula rasa*, reporting and noting things down much as a camera might. Without any guiding perspectives there was the sense of looking at everything, yet wondering in bewilderment what exactly was being observed. Eventually, however, distinctions began to emerge between how people used their personal space around the bed, their conversational styles and their interactions with one another, with myself and with other staff.

Qualitative research is nearer to the activity of a painter than a photographer and my experience often resonated with that described by Lomsky-Feder (1996: 239–240), a woman who studied the experience of war amongst Israeli men. She also found that the maintenance of 'strangeness' is a negotiated or contingent affair and describes this schematically as falling either into the denial of strangeness (reassuring staff that I was not a management 'spy'), the acceptance of strangeness (I was not just another qualified nurse who could be left with the keys) and the presence of strangeness (this refers more to qualities of the researcher, such as a willingness not to instantly accept events at face value, a desire to understand, a recognition of their own 'otherness' and the ability to tolerate a 'marginal' status).

If the ward was particularly busy it could be hard to remember that I was a supernumerary member of staff whose primary function (where ethically acceptable) was to collect research data. The conventional nurse's uniform is generally a tapestry of insignia: colour of dress/shirt, hat, fob watch, pens, badges, scissors on a chain, a mini light for shining in eyes and for senior staff, of course, the keys. Although this paraphernalia was kept to the very minimum at St Christopher's, I felt the need for a visual indicator of my own 'strangeness', a reminder to other staff that I was not a 'real' nurse. I decided to keep the dictaphone in a small pouch around my waist. This apparently small gesture was extremely pointed for a profession that adheres closely to codes of dress and was a powerful symbol of 'otherness'. As a further indicator of my autonomy I would also sometimes leave a shift early or take longer breaks. With participant observation, there is always a danger of entirely 'going native' and the continuous negotiation of role is a tiring balancing act that can sometimes be lonely and disorientating (Sapsford and Abbott 1992).

Sometimes patients seemed to welcome the fact that although I was like the other nurses I was also different. A few asked quite detailed questions about the research, even embarking upon narratives I would only have expected to gather through interviewing. This did not feel like a 'back door' approach to data collection but served to underline Soelle's (1975) conviction that people need to tell their story. Of course, it would have been ethically unacceptable to adopt the persona of an interviewer or to 'steer' conversations towards my own research ends.

While attempting to preserve my researcher identity, I also had to accept that I was entering a new 'language game' (Wittgenstein 1969: paragraphs 19 and 23) where I had to learn the 'rules'. As stranger I could miss certain subtleties, such as the clenched fist of a sleeping woman pointed out to me by her nurse. Even though all the patients were gravely ill, they were never considered to be dying until they reached a particular turning point. Some nurses seemed to recognize this transition almost intuitively, announcing at the shift change, 'Mr Jones is dying now'. Whereas I observed only minimal differences from the previous day, they detected even a slightly diminished level of consciousness, a disturbed breathing pattern or a reduction in urinary output. Sometimes a patient would become restless, plucking at the sheets and unable to settle. Again, this was considered to indicate that the end was imminent. Occasionally, references were made to a recurrent dream or to conversations with deceased relatives. Death would almost invariably follow these signs. If someone rallied, however, the nurses would informally discuss why this might have happened. Could there be a reason for this person to 'hold on'? Were they afraid? They would also review the reasons for their earlier prognosis, searching for any indicators of a flawed original assessment. When those who work in hospice regard actual 'dying' as a relatively brief event characterized by total dependency, I suddenly realized that 'terminally ill people' or 'people approaching death' might have been a more suitable final clauses for the study title. Albeit unconsciously, perhaps the title reflects the way Western culture dramatizes death. It was only as I described manoeuvring a particularly stout fellow into the mortuary fridge one day and noticed the horrified expression of a (non-hospice) friend that I realized the degree to which such incidents are removed from ordinary experience. A new form of life had been entered with different linguistic conventions. It seemed inappropriate, however, to amend anything so fundamental to the procedures of obtaining ethical approval as the study title.

Only once did the desire to observe an incident conflict with my role as carer. In one of the four-bedded bays a man was dying. His family was gathered around the bed praying the rosary. All this was in the direct view of the patient opposite. He repeatedly increased the volume of his television until the room was virtually blasted by the sounds of a popular quiz show. He also placed a number of objects on his bedside table so creating a physical barrier between himself and the scene opposite. As the television decibels rose so did the sound of the prayers. The tension was palpable. This did not feel like the time for a detached observation; the family was more distressed than was strictly necessary. The man 'watching' television clearly required some other distraction. I approached him and asked if he would like to chat for a while. 'No', he responded, 'I'm watching this, I don't want to talk to anyone'. I explained that the volume was rather high and the man opposite was very sick so would he consider watching the programme in the day room? 'No, this is my bed and I won't leave it. I don't think this is at all loud. You're making a fuss about nothing. I don't want to go anywhere else.' Fortunately, at this moment, his wife arrived and within seconds made an accurate appraisal of the situation. She held her husband's hand, took some family photographs from her handbag and gradually drew him into conversation. Within a few minutes she had switched off the television and the rosary opposite faded until it was barely audible. This particular man had witnessed four deaths in his bay. It was hardly surprising if he did not want to 'go anywhere else'; the only place he had observed others depart for was the mortuary. His territory was clearly marked and he was defending it. This was the first incident of this nature and his wife felt that he had been over-exposed to the deaths of fellow patients: 'it's getting to be too much for him'. She found me in another part of the ward specifically to express her thoughts, anxious that I should understand what she felt was very uncharacteristic behaviour.

The participant observer—indeed anyone working in palliative care— should be as skilled in self-observation as in the observation of others. During my induction period as a new member of staff, for example, I spent time in the day centre wearing my own clothes. This soon made me realize some of the protective functions of uniform. Sitting quietly for a moment, a man came and sat next to me. We exchanged a few pleasantries and then he asked me how long I had been a patient. It had never occurred to me that I would be taken as anyone other than a member of staff and, for a split second, I felt off balance and a slight sense of panic. I realized I had been using the sense of being 'other' (staff and not patient) as a defence against certain primitive fears of death. These had to be acknowledged if I was to be able to really observe and listen to patients without erecting obstructions.

To participate on a ward where in some weeks there might be as many (or more) as three deaths, three bodies to lay out and take to the mortuary, three sets of personal possessions to list and pack, three sets of families to comfort, support and assist with practical arrangements, inevitably touches one's own losses and deep feelings concerning mortality. Again, these had to be faced and worked through. There is very little about this affective side of participant observation in the literature, or about the possibility of developing negative feeling towards particular subjects. Once, for example, I registered an apparently quite illogical resistance to one woman. This caused me an immense amount of guilt and self-examination. Eventually, I shared my concern with the ward manager who took a light-hearted view of the matter, 'you don't have to like them to care for them'. Her humour seemed to make caring for and listening to the woman less onerous; the suppression of negative feelings was only locking me into particular perceptions. I decided, therefore, to arrange external supervision from a qualified psychotherapist to help me deal with aspects of my own story that were being invoked by the study. In some fields of research, the need for emotional support can be as great as for academic discussion. Where it is lacking, there may even be an unconscious potential to inflict harm on those whom one is observing or interviewing (Sapsford and Abbott 1992: 127).

There were, however, a number of advantages in becoming immersed in the life of the ward. It provided the opportunity to be with patients throughout the 24-hour cycle. Mornings, evenings and afternoons have different atmospheres and many people expressed their concerns more openly at night. Angela, for instance, was a middle-aged vicar's wife. Each day she was immaculately groomed, confident and poised, entering the kitchen with the air of a volunteer rather than of a patient. At night, however, she would persistently ring her bell and greatly agitated, take her pathology report from her handbag. This she would read aloud, again and again, explaining in tears of disbelief her diagnosis to the nurse on duty. The next morning the report would be neatly folded away and she became 'the vicar's wife' once more. Unable to assimilate the two narratives, Angela suffered their diurnal opposition. A further advantage of working on a ward was that I met virtually every other nurse who worked in the hospice at the various meal breaks, forging a positive rapport that made me less of an unknown factor when I began to visit the wards to recruit volunteers for the interviews.

The interviews

Qualitative research proceeds by inductive rather than deductive logic. It generalizes by abstracting, whereas enumerative induction abstracts by generalization. The process of inference is not the same. In an explorative study such as this, therefore, with stringent ethical safeguards, there was no attempt to establish any randomization of participants. The aim of the study was to provide novel theoretical insights not statistical statements and sampling was purposive. Furthermore, participants were free to converse at whatever level of meaning they felt comfortable. The depth of their response to one of my opening gambits such as 'Can you tell me your story?', 'What brought you here?' or '[How] are you managing to make sense of all this?' lay entirely with the patients. It was noticeable not how few people wanted to talk, but how many and how deeply.

A 'divesting' methodology

Sensitive perceptions sometimes require the suspension of conventional expectation. Although counter intuitive, when listening to terminally ill patients it is important to divest oneself of the notion that the overarching 'happening'—their dying—is the worst thing that could ever happen.

Although most participants clearly regarded their death as catastrophic, for some, when considered against other crises, this was not the case. Irene, for example, regarded the walk out of her first husband, leaving her with three small children, as *the* traumatic incident of her life. Reflecting upon the marriage break-up gave her experience of terminal illness a new perspective. This reinforced her sense of being able to cope: 'I've handled my diagnosis now. Would I have done, before he left me? Probably not … I changed at that point. I won't say I grew up, but my outlook was completely changed. I was the one making the decisions.'

Josie's recurrent depression caused her more anguish than the knowledge of her terminal cancer: 'I've never uttered the words "Why me?" Why not me, if one in three of us get it? But I must say this, it'll say cancer on my death certificate, but so far as I'm concerned, severe depression killed me because it robbed me, of me. It robbed me of my thought processes, I stopped loving music, I became paranoid, I stopped living.' For Judith the thought of further invasive treatment was the more terrifying prospect: 'The surgeon said it was a tumour again, but too deep and difficult for him to operate. But I didn't want another operation. Things looked so awful, that death didn't seem so bad.' Similarly, Irene decided 'No I just can't take it [that is, further treatment]. Had I been younger, or with children at home, I may have for their sake, but my youngest is 34. I made this decision without even telling my husband because I was only an hour away from putting in the Hickman line [an infusion route for delivering chemotherapy]. I just said "I don't want it".' Finally, Camilla expresses the deepest fear of many patients—not the prospect of death itself, but of dying and suffering alone: 'At the end of the day, you are on your own. That really is the bottom line. People can be so kind but really they have no idea what you are feeling like inside and why you are doing what you are doing. It really is the crux of it all—you're on your own.'

Old age may not only bring loneliness, but also the pain of multiple bereavements. When he learned his son was dying from skin cancer, Bernard had already witnessed the death of his alcoholic daughter. Gregory's wife, suffering from dementia, was unable to recognize him. This sorrow he matched, not with the knowledge he was terminally ill, but with his encroaching blindness and inability to make sense of the changes in his life: 'I've had my share of tears, with the wife. When someone you love is slowly disintegrating in front of you, its very emotional. It's all difficult because there is no reason to understand why, is there?'

This early observation of the counter intuitive—that some events can be more traumatic than even that of one's own death, was a valuable lesson. It indicates how easily expectation (dying *must* be the worst thing) can potentially bar one from hearing what is actually being said. More than once, I felt the most important thing I brought to the interviews was not my questions, but my silence. In the words of Suzuki Roshi , 'Usually when you listen to some statement, you hear it as a kind of echo of yourself. You are actually listening to your own opinion' (Longaker 1997: 147). Slowly, I began to learn that to really hear another is akin to an active divestment of self.

Sample profile

A total of 25 people were interviewed: seven men and 18 women. Four people were interviewed more than twice: three women who were still alive 3 months after their initial interview and a man who wanted to add to his original statement. Two of these women were still alive 10 months after their first interview and were interviewed once again. Figures 3.1 and 3.2 illustrate the age and gender distribution of participants. Women were aged from 30 years to 83 years with an average age of 55 years. The men's ages ranged from 49 years to 83 years with an average age of 68 years. All participants were Caucasian, apart from one woman who came to England from the West Indies as a child. A Pakistani woman agreed to take part but, unfortunately, her deterioration prevented her from participating. Interestingly, Jamilla was reluctant to talk as an in-patient, but repeatedly invited me to her home for a meal. I wondered whether this reflected a culturally determined perception of where intimate

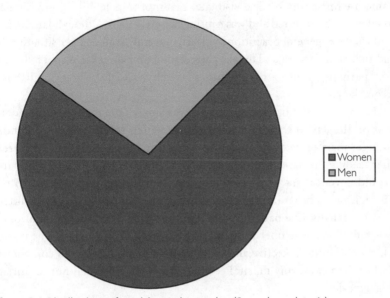

Figure 3.1 Distributions of participants by gender. (See colour plate 1.)

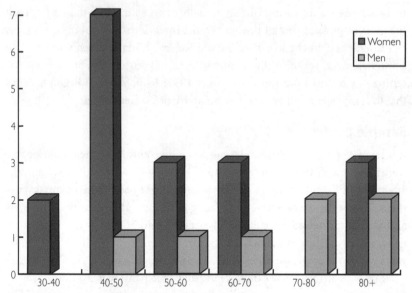

Figure 3.2 Distribution of participants by age and by gender. (See Colour Plate 2.)

conversations should occur. When I telephoned her at home to arrange my visit, however, she sounded rather tearful and her command of English seemed far less secure. Certain that something was wrong, I contacted her homecare nurse who made a visit later that morning. Jamilla's right hip had spontaneously fractured and was causing her great pain. Although Jamilla had contacted her general practitioner, clearly not fully realizing her situation he had advised her to rest and to take paracetamol for pain relief. A sober illustration, perhaps, of the extra difficulties faced by those for whom English is a second language.

The number of participant refusals was small. One man withdrew consent on the day of the interview because he felt too ill to proceed and a younger man agreed when his nurse mentioned the study, but withdrew after reading the patient information form. Another man withdrew because I could never satisfactorily convince him that I was not connected with a BBC television programme being filmed at the same time that I was interviewing. Finally, one patient's wife told the nurse who initially mentioned the study that she felt her husband was too weak to participate. The nurses felt she was over-protective and that he probably would want to contribute. Rather than cause any marital conflict, however, I decided not to pursue this interview.

External influences

Whilst I was recruiting participants, black and ethnic minority patients were also being approached to take part in another piece of qualitative research. People from these social groups are severely under-represented at St Christopher's. Consequently, my fellow researcher and I agreed that I would not approach anyone who might be suitable for her study. For a period of about 6 weeks there was another sense in which the field of enquiry was 'contaminated'. The BBC decided to make an hour-long television documentary about the experience of dying. During this time, I felt as though every patient who might have been a suitable candidate for this study was taking part in the documentary, or had been approached to take part. Some patients seemed to find it difficult to distinguish between the research and the documentary and were clearly suspicious of being involved in the programme. One patient was furious, however, determined to take part in the research simply because it was independent of the programme, protesting 'They make me sick those people. They're like bloody ghouls … riding on our backs and making entertainment out of our misery. It's not right, it's just not right, and it shouldn't be allowed.'

Everyone I interviewed after the film was screened wanted to discuss the programme. When I arrived mid-morning at Josie's home for her interview, her 15-year old daughter, Louise, opened the door and immediately began to cry. Upset by a young man's death, as described by his wife on the programme, Louise did not want to go to school because she wanted to stay near her mother. Deep fears were also triggered for Jane, who suffered from motor neurone disease. Of one patient featured in the film she commented 'Oh, he was fighting, he was really clinging on. It made me feel so sad. When it's my turn, will I fight to stay? I wouldn't want to … but I wonder if the natural instincts just take over? I must admit this worry about suffocation has been on my mind. There's nothing worse than not being able to get your breath. What if you're lying there in a coma, how do they know you're not suffering?' Clearly, when finding potential interviewees in such an agitated state, it is inappropriate to rigidly and insensitively stick to any pre-established process of data collection. It may be kinder and wiser to simply listen without any view to 'getting this down on paper' and to offer appropriate support, in this instance, from a member of the medical team with whom Jane could discuss her anxieties. By demonstrating flexibility and disinterest in her own ends, a researcher is far more likely to establish the trust wherein fears will be safely aired in the future and to be regarded as someone to whom it is 'safe' to refer patients.

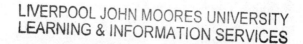

Gender bias?

I visited the wards most days to ask doctors, nurses, physiotherapists and social workers whether there had been any recent admissions who might be suitable for the study. Most of the referrals came from ward nurses, although social workers and homecare nurses also suggested participants. Clearly, far more women were referred to the study than men and those men who were referred were older and nearer to death. Given that 24 beds were reserved for men—a designated capacity nearly 20% greater than the number of beds reserved for women (20)—and that in 1995, 309 women died at the hospice in comparison to 338 men, the ratio of men to women in the study is decidedly low. For some time I purposively tried to recruit more men, yet without any greater success—an experience that is entirely consistent with that of other qualitative researchers in palliative care (Heaven and Maguire 1996).

There are a number of hypotheses for the uneven gender distribution of the study population. Firstly, perhaps equal numbers of men and women were told about the study but men were reluctant to take part. This scenario, however, seems unlikely as staff rarely suggested a man as a potential candidate. This may have been appropriate if staff were correct in judging that fewer men than women wanted to talk about themselves. Significant gender differences in patterns of confiding have been observed elsewhere with men more likely to confide in one person, such as their wife, while women sustain a wider circle of people to whom they speak intimately (Harrison et al. 1995). Similarly, in a study of testicular cancer (Moynihan et al. 1998) most participants did not want to take part in a randomized trial of adjuvant psychological therapy. Clearly, I am not the only researcher to find that men need encouragement to talk.

If the cancers that attack men are more aggressive than those suffered by women, perhaps this accounts for the imbalance in the study population. The period between diagnosis and death would have been shorter for the men, possibly restricting their degree of emotional adjustment. Telling their story may have seemed more of a threat than an opportunity. Although 6 months after interview, six of the seven men were dead (86%) and 10 of the 18 women (56%), figures supplied by St Christopher's admissions office showed no significant gender differences in the average length of in-patient stay. Similarly, a retrospective study of admissions of less than 48 hours (9.8%), covering a 6-month period, did not show a gender bias, although breathlessness was the most frequently reported symptom leading to admission (Boyd 1993).

Stereotypically, women are the carers in our society. A female spouse, daughter or partner might try to keep a sick male relative at home for as long as possible, only supporting his admission when he became too difficult to nurse. At this point, he would probably seem a less likely candidate for research. Information from the *Family Resources Survey for Great Britain* (1994–95: Chapter 6), however, shows that although women do provide most care and younger women provide substantially more than younger men, after the age of 60 there is little difference in their care hours. Higginson *et al.* (1998: 353) demonstrate that, as well as older men and women being less likely to die at home than younger people, men are more likely to die at home than women. Unsurprisingly, social factors significantly influence where patients die. Homecare, for example, may not be available in poorer areas (Higginson *et al.* 1999:22). Hinton (1994: 205) argues that although living alone makes hospice admission more likely, social factors lose something of their significance once a patient comes under the aegis of a homecare team (as was the case for most participants in this study). Clearly, any uni-dimensional hypothesis addressing factors affecting hospice admission or their potential influence on the ratio of men to women in qualitative research must be approached cautiously.

Hospice is a model of care founded by a woman on feminine principles of nurture and support and the majority of carers in hospice are women. Men and women have different styles of communication (Gilligan 1993) and the one-to-one conversation may feel culturally alien to many men. Mentioning the study to men may have been difficult for those I relied upon to introduce me to patients. In an interesting parallel, markedly fewer men are referred to St Christopher's bereavement service than women. Interestingly, during the summer months, I noticed that male smokers seemed to congregate naturally in the garden, creating their own informal 'club'. This model of conviviality perhaps more accurately reflects masculine patterns of self-expression.

It is interesting that men who were referred were older. For one nurse it was easier to care for this age group because she felt they were 'easier to mother'. Occasionally, some of the language used by nurses to describe older men was distinctly emasculating: 'He's such a sweetie/poppet/lamb.' This might suggest that a subliminal sexual ambiguity inhibited younger female carers from mentioning the study to certain men. Certainly, whenever a young man's wife or girlfriend was a regular or constant visitor, the nurses consciously tried not to 'take over'. This reservation suggests some sense of 'trespass' in the nurses' role that might extend to a female researcher. Alternatively, perhaps I was referred more women near to my own age simply because it was assumed that a rapprochement would be easier to establish.

Finally, my own gender may have discouraged some men from participating and it is possible that I subconsciously suggested to staff, despite my overt attempts to recruit more men, that I preferred talking to women. I was certainly more experienced in dealing with sensitive issues with women from my previous employment. It seems likely, however, that the gender imbalance in this and other studies reflects the complexity of the experiences of men and women suffering from terminal illness. An exhaustive exploration lies beyond the parameters of this book and can only be suggested for further research.

Recruitment procedures

I was looking for patients who were aware of the implications of their diagnosis. They were not required to be religious in any formal (or informal) sense, but they did have to feel comfortable talking about their situation. My only exclusion criterion was a history of mental illness. An explanatory leaflet was passed to patients whom carers thought might make suitable participants. If someone was interested in contributing, I would visit to explain the study, only approaching for formal consent 24 hours later if the patient was still keen. The interview could then proceed in another 24 hours' time. These were all necessary ethical safeguards, but each multiplied ten-fold the effort required before an interview could take place. I seemed to be constantly trekking back and forth to the wards trying to strike a happy balance between not being a nuisance yet, despite the welter of all their other work, keeping the research on the nurses' agenda. Inevitably, there were days when the study ranked low priority or the only time the nurse was free to introduce me, the patient was entertaining visitors (I felt it was ethically unacceptable to disrupt these gatherings) or was being sick, was asleep, was on the toilet, was having their dressings tended, had gone out for the afternoon, had just taken medication that influenced their ability to participate, was in the middle of watching a favourite television programme, was waiting for a telephone call, was busy in the day centre, was with their solicitor, was having physiotherapy, was booked to see a social worker, was waiting for the chaplain and so forth. It can be a fallacy that seriously ill people are not busy. The hitches, delays and disappointments seemed to be innumerable and a small number of people died before reaching the stage of the interview. When pain control is very good it is easy to forget just how ill some patients are—deterioration can be rapid and 'unexpected'.

It took a little while for me to appreciate that working in palliative care requires an acceptance of the uncertainty and an inherent unreliability of any study schedule I might establish. It was important to feel calm and relaxed with patients so I always tried to meditate for a few minutes before each interview, which simply means breathing gently and calmly 'collecting' myself in a quiet environment. This was undoubtedly beneficial. I always felt that my ability to listen was diminished when I failed to do this and the patients also seemed to be less forthcoming and relaxed. Sometimes it was difficult to find a suitable venue for the interview, particularly if the patient was in a four-bedded bay with only linen curtains as a barrier. I usually managed to book the day room or an empty side room somewhere. Again, this took a lot of negotiation and careful planning could fall through at the last minute. It was important, however, to create an atmosphere where people could freely enter 'narrative time' without any fear of intrusion, distraction or an embarrassing display of emotion. As one elderly man explained, 'I am happy to do this, and I want to, but it must be somewhere completely private. I couldn't bear it if anyone saw me cry, and I know that I will.' I always had a glass of water, discretely placed tissues and a buzzer to call assistance wherever the interviews were held.

Nobody, however, became uncontrollably upset—although tears were sometimes shed. Of the 25 participants, only three people cried. In each case, this occurred within moments of the interview commencing. It was as though feelings had been suppressed to such a degree that when there was space for their ventilation they burst forth. These people were calm by the end of the interview and expressed gratitude for the opportunity to talk. Two asked whether I could visit again, one of whom sent for me a few days later because he wanted to 'talk some more'. My role, however, was that of researcher, not therapist or counsellor. Although I did spend some more time with this man, once it was clear that no new data were emerging, I suggested he might like to meet the chaplain or a social worker. A few days later, I called in briefly again; I did not want him to feel abandoned or rejected because of any self-disclosures made during our conversations. Nearly all the interviewees were seen again socially for this reason and also to thank them. I was especially punctilious about this where participants took up my offer of either hearing their tape or of reading its transcript. Words given in passing acquire a solidity and solemnity in text. It seemed plausible to imagine a patient traumatized by reading thoughts on illness and death, even if they had provided them verbally. Sadie, for example, recoiled at seeing her condition in print: 'The other day, my husband brought me a letter from the council. It said I was seriously ill. I didn't like seeing it in black and white. ... He said, "No one else sees it", so I said back, "Well, you're not it, are you?" Much as he cares, much as it's crippling him, I'm the one at the sharp end and it's no good.' Most people, however, were pleased with their transcripts, commenting on parts they liked or found surprising. Josie's response was typical: 'I've said it, so it must be true and I'll stand by it.' Amusingly, when Hazel read her transcript she sent for me 'urgently'. Alarmed, I hurried to see her. Always particular, she had noticed one or two typing errors and did not want me to 'get into trouble'. She seemed calm and pleased with her contribution. Humbled, I took this on face value.

More challengingly, Josie asked if she could keep her tape for a couple of weeks to listen to with her children aged 15 and 23 years. This unanticipated request caused me some disquiet. I had ethical reservations. The interview had been a private discussion and, although support could have been quickly arranged through the social work department, there was no way I could know how her offspring would respond to the tape. This incident also raises the issue of the ownership of data. Does a tape 'belong' to the study participant, especially if it concerns biographical details, or to the researcher? Much has been made of this issue in the ethics protocols of collaborative research but I had not foreseen circumstances where a participant might use the research experience as a means to another end, in this instance, inter-family communication. I decided to take the philosopher Ricoeur's line on the 'ownership' of text. He argues that although the written (and presumably recorded) word may not be entirely disassociated from its author's intended meaning, the association is sufficiently distended for text to have a life of its own. Even with an old or familiar text, fresh disclosures are always possible and the passage of time brings new associations. Thus, there is a sense in which none of us can exercise ownership, in the sense of total control, over our words. I allowed Josie to keep the tape, which she returned saying it had been 'very helpful'. Perhaps Josie was simply more frank than other participants. Once they were released to interviewees, I had no means of knowing what they did with their transcripts or tapes.

Motivational factors

The reasons why people took part in the research gradually emerged as multiple. Some freely admitted that they were bored and it was useful to have something to pass the time. Others emphasized their pleasure at 'doing something for the hospice'. One or two used the time to achieve unrelated goals. Arthur, for example, was being considered as suitable for discharge to a nursing home. He clearly regarded his interview as a prime opportunity to argue against this: 'I don't want to go, I don't need to go. I like it here. I feel secure here.' He had also asked for his stepdaughter to be present at the interview. No one was to be in any doubt about his feelings on this matter.

Interestingly, Arthur was one of only three participants, two men and one woman, who asked for someone else to be present during their interview. For both men this was established when they consented to participate. Fred was a 49-year-old administrator who died only five days after his interview and although he proclaimed 'My wife and I are a unit; there's not a thing she doesn't know about me; we're two bodies but one in spirit', I felt that he began to use our conversation to address himself less to myself than to Janice, his wife. It became a vehicle for him to express great tenderness and concern and to demonstrate a realistic, yet masculine 'fighting' attitude, all in the guise of a factual statement: 'I want to live, I'll try me best to live. My material worries are over, barring one, which is Janice hasn't passed her driving test yet. But once she's done that she's fully mobile. All the house papers and everything are in order and she's got money in the bank and that's a relief to me. You see, I've got such a love for Janice, I didn't want any messes left behind me. In that respect, I'm quite happy.'

I had not expected two of Tracey's children, 9-year-old Jack and 12-year-old Laura, to be at home when I called. I was unsure about how much the children knew of their mother's situation and was treading rather gingerly until they left the room to fetch some tea and biscuits. I expressed my concerns to Tracey, suggesting that even though she might not feel inhibited by their presence, it was possible for memories or events to surface during the course of her interview that she might want to withhold if the children could hear. Tracey, the veteran of 12 major abdominal operations, was emphatic in her response: 'Even my youngest one knows everything. He's nine and he knows as much as what I know. And that's quite a lot. Most people say "Oh, you should hide it from them", but I'm being straight. They accepted it better. If I only told them half, they would be wondering about the rest. They know if anyone comes round, or doctors, I'd never leave them out. The kids know that. "That's it, innit Laura? You're always in on the conversation." They see everything that happens to me, they're there with me' (by now the children had returned with a tray).

For Tracey, no children meant no conversation. Although she justified their presence in terms of conforming to her existing pattern of dealing with professionals, I also sensed that she found their presence supportive. She clearly depended on her children for motivation, emotional sustenance and protection, continuing 'My husband blanks it totally. Can't accept it, won't speak about it. Makes it harder for me ... but, lucky enough, I've got the kids. As I said, my Jack [the nine year old], he knows more about me than my husband. It's really weird because he's a normal kid playing about, but as soon as there's a doctor in the house, he's watching, looking, asking questions. Jack would defend, stand in front and say "Leave my mum alone." He won't let anything happen to me. Nobody can talk about me. No one can touch me and if I need anything he's the one who gets it.'

At this point in our conversation, Jack and Laura were ostensibly watching television. Laura sat on the floor and Jack was leaning against his Mum on the settee. He was still in his school uniform and fingering a Christmas decoration he had made earlier. He seemed a little uncertain about my presence and after the following exchange it felt appropriate to interrupt Tracey's comments:

Tracey: You know about Mummy's illness?

Jack: Yeah …?

Tracey: Do you think I should tell you or not tell you about it? Do you think I should hide it from you or tell you about it?

Jack: Tell me about it.

Tracey: Why?

Jack: Just in case Dad goes out and you're ill or something, I won't know what to do.

Tracey: That's right.

Jack was looking worried, as though he suspected something was afoot. Although the purpose of my visit had been explained, some reassurance was clearly required so I said 'That's very sensible. Your Mum asked because I've come from St Christopher's and we've been talking about everything. Nothing has changed; we've just been talking about it. Nothing has changed.' Jack was clearly relieved and I expected the 'interview' to wind down, but Tracey suddenly took the initiative, seizing the moment to establish and affirm her own priorities. With an urgency and imperative she turned to Jack, 'You know what to do if Mummy dies don't you? You know what I want? What stone I want? You know all that?' For Jack, however, this seemed to be a conversation familiar almost to the point of boredom:

Jack: What stone? Oh yeah, a heart one.

Tracey: A heart stone but you know I'm not gonna be there [pointing to the ground]. Where am I going to be?

Jack: [sitting upright with a grin and hitting his chest] Near me!

Tracey: Floating … like that [indicating with her hand]. Floating near you, near Laura.

Jack: [grinning and teasing] You best not scare me, Mummy. If you do, I'll scream.

Tracey: No, I won't scare you, but I'll never leave you, will I?

Jack: No.

Tracey: [to me] See, they all know this and [to the room, emphatically and rhetorically] it makes us stronger dunnit?

Jack and Laura: Mmmm … yeah.

This conversation was an opportunity for Tracey to reinforce her preparation of her children for her death, to display her fortitude and to demonstrate her 'good mothering'. From her point of view, it was worthwhile and at the end she leaned back with obvious satisfaction. Her attitude brings to mind the work of Baruch (1981) who reveals how mothers of disabled children tell stories which appeal to their 'responsibility' in the face of adversity. Clearly, interview responses are not simply accurate (or otherwise) *reports* on reality, but can be '*displays* of perspectives and moral forms' (Silverman 1994: 107). To dispel some of the preceding intensity, before I left, Jack, Laura and I played with the tape recorder creating 'interviews' of our own and generating much laughter. As I walked up the garden path, Jack ran after me with one of his chocolates from the Christmas tree and the injunction to 'keep it for later if you're not hungry now'.

This interview illustrates one of the many potential transformations of a researcher's identity that may be wrought by a study participant. I was promoted to the status of the reliable witness; someone to whom Tracey could demonstrate her love for her children and her concern for their future. In other interviews I felt there were moments when my status became that of confidante (by those who spoke of love affairs or sexual relationships), of confessor with the ability to dispense forgiveness (by at least two men who spoke of their war-time activities), of comforter or even of judge (one woman lamented throughout 'I could have done better. I could have tried harder'). Perhaps the fact that I did not wear a uniform for this stage of the study made my relationship to patients less defined and therefore more open to transmutation. People often commented on how busy the doctors and nurses seemed and how hard they had to work. Perhaps because I did not present as a 'real' worker with other important duties it was easier for patients to slide into conversation without feeling guilty or greedy for 'taking too much time'.

Conducting an interview in the patient's own home gave a broader access to their world, their particular time frame and their pace of living. On another occasion, an interesting conversation arose when Tracey asked me if I would stay for a while to watch the Wimbledon tennis with her. We both sat drinking tea with our feet up. When an advertisement for some beauty product was screened, it prompted Tracey to express thoughts about her altered body and how she felt: 'a lot of people don't like me anymore. I'm so outspoken since I've been ill. I can't be bothered with pretences.' Perhaps because patients are so often the recipients of care, they seem to enjoy proffering hospitality. Watching tennis was something 'normal' and, I hope, made Tracey feel she was valued for her own sake as much as for her research contributions. In a goal-driven culture, 'wasting' time sometimes requires a certain moral courage, but simply watching television, helping with some knitting, or other generally undirected activities can bring multiple insights and cement a trusting rapport.

Being in someone's home placed conversations in context. Ornaments, colours, photographs and so forth all provided valuable cues and points of reference. These interviews were generally longer and people seemed more relaxed. It was also possible to make supportive observations. Jane, for example, had mentioned that although her partner David cared, he could never talk to her: 'He bottles things up—can't face it.' When David arrived home for an unexpected break from his job as a van driver, before he entered the room I offered to leave. Jane said this was not necessary; we could all take a break together. David, however, took his tea and a newspaper into the lavatory and remained there until he left for work again. Sighing, Jane explained how this was his typical behaviour when the homecare nurses called: 'It's just how he is. He doesn't want to hear or be reminded, it's all too much for him.'

In other interviews there were moments when it seemed necessary to 'permit' the less socially acceptable subtext to surface, to intimate that latent tears or swearing were not censorious. Carla, a 49-year-old mother of three teenage boys, was a long-term patient at the hospice. Metastases from her breast cancer had caused her leg to spontaneously fracture and she was confined to her bed. The atmosphere in her room was heavy and Carla seemed to exhale her cigarette smoke in a somewhat defiant manner. Our conversation proceeded thus:

Interviewer: How are you feeling?

Carla: Oh, not too good really, I feel …

Interviewer: Mmm?

Carla: [pause] Pretty bad [looking very fed up].

Interviewer: Are you being restrained? … Do you feel like putting it more strongly?

Carla: [slowly and with emphasis] Yes, I feel like a fucking shit bag. That's how I feel. Nothing but a fucking shit bag.

We both grinned at this and the way seemed open for a frank conversation. More than once I felt the focus of powerful feelings of loss, anger or even of misplaced affection. The external supervision I had arranged was of inestimable value in helping to recognize elements possibly connected with the phenomena of transference, counter-transference or projective identification (Dalley 1989: 11). I realized, for example, that my use of 'restraint' in the above exchange was almost certainly influenced by the fact Carla's leg was in traction. This traction was very similar to that used on my own sister, Charlie, after the excision of a tumour when we were children. Note the similarity of the pseudonym I selected for 'Carla'. Without the safeguard of the supervision, the potential for subconscious projections was high. Powerful and inappropriate feelings easily surface in vulnerable people (and interviewers) when sensitive subjects are discussed intimately. At least one patient was embarrassed and confused by the depth of affection she had developed for her social worker: 'I feel so stupid. Like a kid, a teenager, but I'm feeling really in love. It's stupid but I think about him all the time. I can't help myself. I'd die if he knew but I want to know *everything* about him.'

It was not always easy to gauge the significance attached by patients to particular aspects of their narrative; the apparently inconsequential point, such as the forgotten place name, could sometimes seem a tremendous stumbling block. I had to learn to be patient, relinquishing any desire to 'move' the interview on to what I thought 'really' mattered. Convictions such as 'I was here', 'I did this' or 'I used to count' were buried in the salvaged dates and places. They explain the intensity of Arthur's response to my unwitting insensitivity in an early interview:

Arthur: Growing up, I was in a ... er ... a convalescence home ... They sent me to a convalescence home ... if I can just remember the name ... er ... [pause]

Interviewer: It doesn't matter if you can't remember the name.

Arthur: [loudly and with feeling] It *does* ... It does matter to *me*.

After this, I decided only to approach people for consent when there were few other patients within earshot. I did not want to raise questions and insecurities such as 'Why didn't she ask me?', 'Why have I been left out?', 'Isn't my story worth hearing?' or 'Don't I matter?'.

It is not only the identity and function of an interviewer that is contingent. The self-presentation of participants is also open to negotiation. Miller (1996: 141) draws attention to a potential ethical dilemma. Perhaps, simply by taking part in an interview, patients feel under some pressure to change or to present a particular 'world view'. Carla once suggested that perhaps she failed to meet some imaginary standard of interest by asking 'Is this the type of answer you are looking for, or do you want something more outstanding? I sometimes think that I'm rambling. I don't want to because you've got a tape. I don't want to waste it'.

If Carla felt she should offer 'more' for her story to be worth hearing, Bernard's interview became an act of persuasion rather than of description; an opportunity for him to reclaim a measure of potency and agency more typical of his earlier life. In a study of middle-aged businessmen, Ochberg (1987) focuses on how each man describes the development of his career, concluding that the telling of each story is a symbolic bridge connecting with what was *not* said about the relationships of these men with their father. Interestingly, Bernard used the early part of his interview to present himself as the successful businessman of his earlier years, taking out his diary to confirm particular dates, wearing a shirt and tie and questioning me about specific aspects of data collection, academic supervision and data analysis. This was a far cry from his distress as he described the break-up of his relationship with his girlfriend, the death of his daughter and his son's recent diagnosis of a malignant condition. Until his narrative became more personal, he had been very much in control, very much the executive. Suddenly his story took a twist, invoking the image of a mountain. This was clearly 'unsafe ground' and Bernard rather formally, but abruptly, excused himself from the room:

> Bernard: … Hillary … he was the man who conquered Everest … [voice fading, almost talking to himself]
>
> Interviwer: [sounding surprised at this apparently unrelated thought] Oh, Edmund Hillary … yes?
>
> Bernard: I often think about things to make my mind consider … [pause]
>
> Interviwer: [quietly] Consider … ?
>
> Bernard: [briskly] Well, I must love you and leave you then.

The mountain is a symbol with an ancient heritage and its intrusion into the safety of a persuasive narrative will be unsurprising to those familiar with images resulting from deep unconscious material (Stewart 1996). Bernard also expressed profound fears for the future and felt he was an 'obstacle' to the happiness of others: 'I sometimes think it might be a good thing if I just went away.' When discourse enters this territory of symbolism and imagery, what Fromm (1951) calls the 'forgotten language', the researcher is presented with an interpretive challenge and any derivative theoretical statements require large numbers of supportive data and sound literary references. The notion of a narrative subtext is troubling. It suggests that, for some reason, the narrator is unable to tell their own story. 'This seems especially demeaning when our informants have been oppressed; here listening to an account on any terms but those on which it is offered seems like an act of further disenfranchisement' (Ochberg 1996: 98). It is naïve, however, to assume that people always say what they mean and mean what they say. Bernard and Angela—the vicar's wife mentioned earlier—demonstrate how social codes and personal censorship will influence the tenor and content of an interview. Each was committed to a self-image they felt obliged to defend. Although Bernard's need to exercise control dominated his interview, in a rare moment of openness he admitted of this behaviour: 'Well, really and truly, it's all a masquerade. All I'm doing is hiding myself away from people and not letting them know what is wrong with me. I don't want to expose myself as a sick or inferior person. I don't want people to see that I am as I am.'

Shift of focus

The decision to discontinue recruitment was made when a saturation level seemed to have been reached and unfamiliar or new insights were no longer emerging. Honouring this cut-off point requires a resolute ability to resist making one more interview 'just in case'. Qualitative research, however, is not about making statistically significant statements. A large and cross-matched study cohort is not required for a study to make useful and penetrative insights. The cut-off point demonstrates a conviction that sufficient data have been gathered to construct a credible 'new' story. When data collection and analysis are as intertwined as in this study, any transfer of attention from one to the other is less a juncture than a transition with broad overlap.

Chapter 4

A story in the making: data analysis and interpretation

Introduction

To analyse or to interpret data is to tell a new story. A natural tension exists between this telling and the desire to remain loyal to the original material upon which it relies. To tell a story about another is partly about wielding power. There is always a danger of making that frightening step to where 'there is no need to hear your voice when I can talk about you better than you can talk about yourself' (Fine 1994: 70). Consequently and as far as possible, patients' own words resonate throughout this exploration of their spiritual needs. Any novel theoretical insights are firmly grounded in the metaphors by which they lived and died.

There are those who argue that qualitative researchers should 'bracket out' any preconceptions they may hold about their field of enquiry (Husserl 1962). 'Bracketing' supposedly prevents the intrusion of 'bias' and defends the objectivity of interpretation. Of course, some degree of self-consciousness is crucial to the sensitive conduct of research, but 'immaculate perception' is an impossible goal. 'Answers' are framed by the structure of questions and 'questions' presuppose a complex matrix of cultural and cognitive factors. By choosing to focus on one subject, we inevitably exclude others from the frame of enquiry. All researchers' perceptions are historically and culturally located and it is impossible to exclude 'taken for granted' knowledge. Indeed, without it, distinguishing a patient's 'knowing look' from a blank gaze is impossible. This reasoning follows the philosopher Heidegger (1962) on what he called the 'hermeneutic circle' with its argument that consciousness is always consciousness of something and his consequent disavowal of 'uninterpreted facts'. For understanding to occur, this 'circle' must be entered, but it is only entered through understanding. There is no place 'outside' the circle from which to impartially observe, analyse or interpret events. Although this cycle is logically unbreakable, it is fractured each time a new understanding occurs—bringing to mind the image of a spiral, perhaps, more than that of a circle. It is the constant revision of focus between parts and whole that allows new understandings of the two to emerge. Understanding is thus a matter of participation and knowledge is no longer approached in foundational terms, but in terms of its practicality. Does it work? Is it helpful? Is it applicable to this time and situation? Any notion of providing a 'final word' on a subject is an oppressive ideal, reminiscent of Enlightenment ideals.

None of this, however, means that 'anything goes' for the qualitative researcher. The conditions for achieving reliability, taken as identical repetition, may be available only to the natural sciences (and there not without some qualification), but notions of 'audit' provide an alternative standard of rigour in qualitative research (Guba and Lincoln 1981). Memoranda, field notes, accurate interview transcriptions and records of compliance and refusal trace the logic of this study of spirituality in terminally ill people from the development of its protocol to its interpretive criteria and sense of ethical responsibility.

Processes of analysis and interpretation may be indissoluble, but they are subtly distinctive. Many studies focus on the analytical (from the Greek to loosen or untie) at the expense of consideration of the interpretive (from the Latin to explain the meaning of something). This has perhaps contributed to a superficial understanding of what is involved in creating a 'new story', shoring up a confidence in the infallibility of immediate appearances and a conviction that if a set of data is sufficiently broken into its constituent parts it will eventually 'speak for itself' (Cowman 1993). The ideal however, is a deft analytical handling of data that is open to the pluri-potential of interpretation.

The participant observation and over 25 interviews with patients, each of at least 40 minutes' duration, generated literally pages of data. Some flexible and efficient method of handling this material was clearly necessary. Analysis is a struggle between immersing and distancing oneself from raw data, of moving back and forth between conceptual and abstract levels of thought and I decided this would be best facilitated by the NUD*IST (non numerical unstructured data indexing and theorizing) computer programme (Richards and Richards 1993). While, however, the computer is a priceless analytical tool (simultaneously creating an 'audit trail'), it is not an agent of interpretation. Computers ultimately treat text as numbers, as an inherently meaningless collection of representations. A crucial difference between analysis using a computer programme and textual interpretation lies in this fact (Pfaffenberger 1988). Handling data in this manner may precipitate concepts and meanings, but the programme is only ever a tool. It is the researcher who recollects the conditions of data collection and who is aware of the nuances of discourse, or of the 'feeling' of silence.

Expanding possibilities

Painstaking and methodical analysis bears certain comparisons with excavation, with searching for meanings that lie hidden 'behind' data or camouflaged within their inter-relations. Interpretation of a text (where 'text' includes what people say or do), however, is about more than this. It is about the expansion of possibility (Ricoeur 1971, 1981). Interpretation opens up the world in ways that are closed to a strictly thematic or structural analysis. This stance is not opposed to analysis *per se*, but regards it as a potentially reductionist and naïve first step in the understanding of human experience. Meaning is not simply 'hidden' within text. It opens up 'before' text by encouraging us to look at things in a new way, to think in a new manner, to make new connections. This is not about identifying with the mind of the text's 'author' (in no sense, for example, does this book attempt to 'step into the shoes' of its contributors). Rather, text carries an injunction for us to see the world afresh. By so doing, it legitimately refers beyond its own contents and context. This approach is simply another endorsement that life is larger than language, art, analysis or interpretation. It may be that the least inscribable aspect of an event carries the greatest potency. Cox and Theilgaard (1987: 116), in their study of serious offenders, for example, cite a man who murdered his wife: 'She said nothing, so I killed her. Then nothing was said.'

The following brief story, recounted by a homecare nurse, also illustrates how meaning resists total seizure. Three days after a patient's funeral, his wife was sitting quietly at his graveside when a small robin perched by her foot. She found this simple incident profoundly comforting, wanting to 'talk of nothing else' at the nurse's next visit. In the words of the nurse, 'I'm sure she felt this was spiritually significant in some way, but I can't explain how.' Through the idea of all events possessing a 'surplus of meaning', a significance or depth that is literally ungraspable, Ricoeur (1976) accommodates dimensions of reality that extend beyond immediate impressions. To consider the robin as carrying an ultimate as well as human significance is thus a legitimate move. Like many an artistic disclosure, this small incident is not without the potential to make present that which may not be said, so allowing the bereft woman to glimpse far horizons of meaning in the immediacy of the prosaic. Words, in the sense of labelling, are not necessary to convey this type of meaning and Carla's comments seem relevant: 'What can anyone say about my dying? There are no words. But friends don't need words to say what they mean and I can say anything to you now.'

My aim is not to tell the patients' stories better than they can themselves, that would be an abusive distortion. In recounting their words and deeds I try to preserve an openness to possibility, to foster an understanding that different depths of meaning are anchored in the particular and that these depths are never exhaustively fathomed. Furthermore, since, text is 'an object that can be viewed from several sides but never from all sides at once' (Ricoeur 1976: 77), conflicts of interpretation are not only inevitable, but they are to be welcomed as a means of advancing knowledge. Finally, the disclosive potential of the nurse's story demonstrates how 'depth perceptions' are a 'showing that is, at the same time, creating a new mode of being' (Ricoeur 1976: 88). In short, the bereaved woman is altered by her encounter with the robin—as evidenced by her excited talking of it. The following pages attempt a similar 'showing' in that they are partially motivated by a desire to help carers recognize patients' spiritual concerns. Hopefully, in ways that make it possible for them to help another who is searching for somewhere to stand when it seems there is no ground underfoot.

Part 2

Spiritual concerns expressed in non-religious ways

Chapter 5

Features of a 'language of spirit'

Introduction

One of the most perplexing matters facing modern carers is how to recognize when patients are expressing spiritual or ultimate concerns if they are not using religious language. Based on the methodologies described earlier, this chapter tries to identify some of the characteristics or 'tools' of a non-religious (but not necessarily so) language of spirit. When every movement is also a gesture, language (verbal and written) is only one symbol system amongst many. There are myriad and diverse means of human communication and we are interested in any that manifest spiritual concerns. We all can, and often do, say more than we know. For a statement or piece of behaviour to be making some spiritually significant disclosure, therefore, it is not necessary for its perpetrator to be fully aware of its potential. This is not to say that, in trying to understand their words or deeds, we are 'reading anything into' what patients say or do (meaning anyhow emerges in the exchange between a 'text' and its reader). Rather, as argued in the previous chapter, data are better considered in terms of the novel insights that open up before them.

Matrix of 'happenings'

Carol used the term 'happenings' as she mused over the many changes in her life after developing motor neurone disease. It is also a good term for describing the fluid matrix of symbols from which the language of spirit emerges, but which it also constitutes. When considering this language, we are constantly refocusing between its specific 'tools' or characteristics and the language as a thing in itself. This process is a bit like concentrating on the individual knots of a fishing net and then on the net as a whole. We are caught in the tension implicit whenever one thing is said to constitute another, for although there is a sense in which the latter is made from the former 'without remainder', there is also a sense in which it exists as 'more than' that which makes up its parts.

Despite the continuing need to shift between parts and whole, however, it is possible to identify three relatively distinct aspects of a language of spirit: its context, its literary form and its symbolic form. Respectively, these find expression in selective vignettes of behaviour and biographical details: in a configuration of vernacular and archaic language and the use of humour, in the presence of certain permeating themes, emergent symbolic meanings and ancient spiritual motifs and in the use of ritual and silence as expressive media. These three aspects are organizational rather than definitive categories and defy hard-and-fast exclusivities. Paradox, for example, straddles categories of both symbolic and literary form, while silence presents the ambiguities and tensions of the absent presence—the 'tool' that is, but is not, there. Similarly, although the ancient spiritual motif of the mandala is an instantly recognizable literary or visual form, here it is primarily treated as a symbol and is located in a discussion of linguistic structuralism. The main point, however, is that each aspect is sufficiently recognizable to be useful and supports the notion of a language of spirit. On different occasions and contributed by different patients, 'happenings' from each aspect have been used to disclose the possibility of a human and ultimate horizon of meaning.

Language of spirit: context

Although meaning often extends beyond the content and referent of language, the first aspect of a language of spirit acknowledges that language is always about something (even if it expresses an untruth). If it were not contextual, language would just be noise. Failing to acknowledge the varying circumstances of the patients in this study, therefore, or the common 'overarching happening'—their imminent death, would denude any discussions in favour of a language of spirit.

This Chapter and the next (5 and 6) are ideally considered as a pair. Here, we concentrate upon how a language of spirit works and later, upon what patients say about their lives when they use this language. Consequently, the lion's share of contextual information that distinguishes the patients' investigated circumstances from any other personal events is reserved for the following chapter. Nevertheless, in the hope of grounding the comments and remarks that do arise here, Young and Cullen (1996) have been followed and brief monographs of contributing patients (under a pseudonym, of course) are given as an appendix to this chapter. Presenting any profile of another is a delicate matter and although detailed personality 'types', 'stages of acceptance' and specific 'tasks' of living and dying are popular and often helpful approaches in research about the spiritual needs of palliative care patients (Brown and Williams 1993; Cowan 1991; Kellehear 2000; Millison 1995), they are neither used or implied in these vignettes. Such literature effectively organizes observers' perceptions by establishing second-order propositions. This study is distinguishable by its reliance upon the first order—for allowing people their own voice. Staying as close to patients' own words and deeds as possible, the following chapter presents the major metaphors they use to invent (that is, both to create and to discover) their being-in-the-world (Dreyfus 1991; Heidegger 1962). Each metaphor is a miniature 'story' by which patients both live and die. Whilst conceding that there are no uninterpreted facts and that any putting aside of personal convictions may only be relative, this emphasis on the first order also defers the necessity of constructing abstract theoretical frameworks about spirituality.

Language of spirit: literary form

Two specific literary forms of expression are especially characteristic of the language of spirit. Each is valued both for its recognizable structure and its expressive effect. These two forms, archaic language and humour, are not simply matters of communicative style. When used by patients, each form effects its own distinctive and subtle import of meaning in addition to any information it may convey.

Archaic language

The value of careful listening, of stillness and receptivity in times of confusion and of a generally 'divesting methodology' has already been commented upon. These attitudes are perhaps most important for the appreciation of archaic language, whose impact is powerful because 'as deep calls unto deep' (*Psalm* 42, Chapter 7), it touches our depths (Kearney 1992: 45). Although 'archaic language is easy to recognize, it is not easy to define. It is not necessarily "old", in the sense of being written in the remote past or even antiquity. It tends to be condensed, concise, direct, forceful, vivid, inferential and it is affect-laden. It carries existential weight' (Cox and Theilgaard 1987: 139).

Many of the patients were searching for reasons for their illness and frequently invoked metaphors of 'reaping what one sows'. Julia, for instance, wondered whether the occupational stress she always courted had provoked her cancer. For Claude, years of smoking explained his disease. Tracey blamed a more general self-neglect that stemmed from always putting her family first. Sometimes this search, or some other aspect of a patient's experience, was expressed in distinctly archaic terms. At our first meeting, Claude sat, head in hands, poring over a meticulous bank ledger. His desire to 'make things up to my wife before it's too late', his intensity and his interesting mixture of content and cadence—typical of archaic language—all suggest that the gravity of his situation extended far beyond mathematical calculations. Looking up, his words were 'I can't get these to balance and I must before the night falls.'

Reflecting upon their work with schizophrenic patients, Cox and Theilgaard argue that archaic language is 'technically regressive' in that it is a return to an earlier (in the sense of primordial) tongue, but it functions as the opposite of defence because it enables frightening thoughts and feelings to be expressed. They write, 'We can guess, we can infer why archaic language is so frequently invoked to carry our deepest feelings. Yet it is so. And this phenomenon is independent of formal education and degree of literacy. It may have something to do with the point at which "everyday language" breaks down because too much is expected of it' (Cox and Theilgaard 1987: 142). In an interesting correlation with Claude's balancing of accounts, they also associate archaic language with the notion of existential debt, arguing that such debts are often better expressed in a language that is timeless for each generation: 'It may be a debt of gratitude to life, a debt of taking life for granted or a debt evident of some other invisible loyalty' (Cox and Theilgaard 1987: 142). This also pertains to certain notions of 'fairness' invoked by Claude, whose absence of physical pain seemed not to equate with an absence of suffering, but almost to be its source: 'I just have to press a bell and three or four nurses come running … It's not what I deserve. I've been a heavy smoker. I've inflicted this on myself.'

No experience is uninterpreted and phenomena may be regarded not only in terms of 'Why?' but also of 'What for?'. If Claude felt he merited punishment, Fred's illness was a learning experience, 'part of a lesson I've got to learn'. Calamitous events are usually considered in terms of personal import (Cassell 1982: 641), but they often entail a series of wider connections. Mary, for example, 10 days before her death said, 'A lot of people say "don't you ask "Why Me?"" But I believe that God has a plan for me and my family, and it doesn't include me being on this earth anymore. I've reached a point where my life is no longer of any use. I would be sad if I felt fine, very sad, but I don't feel fine.' It is in limit situations such as Mary's, when one finds oneself at the furthest points of human tolerance and understanding, that archaic language tends to emerge, sometimes sounding almost psalmic: 'All the struggles, all the uphill climbs, but my spirit says to me, "stop worrying, occupy yourself"'(Debbie).

Humour

The second literary form characteristic of a language of spirit is that of humour. If 'every story someone tells us is a snapshot of their inner world' (Longaker 1997: 146), humour is a means of safely approaching and disarming the otherwise inexpressibly painful or overwhelming. Amusing anecdotes or comments, even when saturnine, may be 'signals of transcendence'. They may be indicators of ultimate awareness and lead towards a 'theology of the comic' (Berger 1997). Sadie asked if I would like to hear a joke:

> This man goes up to heaven. A guy goes up to him so he says 'What's going on?' The guy says 'Here's the entrance to heaven. Whether or not you take the decision to come in is up to you, but once you've made it, that's it.' This guy's a bit of a joker, a bit of a lad. He opens a door and all these people are up to their ankles in shit. In their hands is a glass of water. The first guy says 'Oh no, I don't want that, don't like that'. 'Fair enough' says the other guy and they go to the next door. All these people are up to their knees in it, but they've got a bottle of beer between them. The guy goes 'No, no, can't be. I can't have that. No, no, no, there's got to be some catch, I'll go on.' So he goes to the last door. Now they're up to their shoulders in it, but they've each got a glass of whisky. The bloke goes 'Well it's not too bad and I suppose you get used to the smell.' So it's 'in you go'. The bloke just goes to step in and the leader of the group says 'Right, you've had your 5 minutes' break. All back on your hands and knees.'

Tightly clenched hands and darting eyes betray a deeper significance to the joke and Sadie naturally transferred the artificial chance to her own situation; 'Well, I haven't got a choice. I'd love it if I had a choice, if I tried really hard so I could be allowed some more time with my husband.' Without wishing to push the comparison too far, the time-honoured comic formula of three options with a twist in the third parallels Sadie's two earlier failed marriages and more recent union. Again, life had not turned out according to Sadie's plan. Her increasing weakness also meant there was no 'let out' even in distracting chores, 'I'd do the ironing, I'd clean the windows every day. I just can't face reality at all … I don't know what's going to happen. [whispering] If someone's dying I can't just walk in and ask … But I don't really want to know either.'

Sadie was sitting tight: 'I don't want to move from where I am. I don't want to know, although I've got to ask, sooner or later.' Her's was a potentially explosive situation, 'sooner or later' something would have to give. Certainly, Sadie was tense, agitated even by the slight whirring of the interview recorder before it was placed on a soft blanket: 'What's that ticking noise? Is it going to blow up, a bomb?' This destructive image re-occurred: 'My parents are lovely, but they sort of coo coo coo [spoken softly and slowly] around me. You see, my dad, he'll sort of run and kiss me in case I go "ch ch ch ch ch" [said in a brisk even staccato] and self-destruct and that's all that's left of me, a handful of rubber, or something.' The onomatopoeic 'ch ch ch' supports the notion of seconds ticking away, the compression of possibility and emphasizes the drama of what was, for Sadie, an only child, an inexplicable inversion: 'I'm very responsible for Mum and Dad. I always knew I would be the one to care for them, now it won't be down to me. It's the other way around. I just can't face it.'

Grace also illustrates how laughter may provide sufficient camouflage to forge an uneasy truce with reality and so 'paper over' existential wonderings. She was a child of seven when, in late Victorian splendour, her deceased father was laid out in the front parlour. Apart from a small chink, the curtains were drawn. The enterprising Grace soon realized that she could charge her friends a penny each to be sneaked, with verve and bravado, through the shrubbery up to the windowsill for a peep. No sooner had she finished laughing at this memory than, *sotto voce*, she recounted a terrifying recurrent nightmare. A tall, cloaked and hooded figure would be walking towards the side of her bed, his face obscured. The moment he reached out to touch her, she would wake, in a cold sweat. Memory and dream are associated for both speak of trepidation before the unknown. Myth and legend assure that few escape to describe death once it has been stared in the face. Even as children, Grace and her friends realized that observation of death is dangerous. The support of friends is required and such an enterprise always extracts a price—one has to pay the ferryman to cross the Styx. Given all this, the human tendency is to screen or 'curtain' death from life. The protective mantle of an amusing childhood reminiscence veils these stark truths, diffusing the power of the unknown night figure by using the same dynamic between participation and distance that permits any feelings of cultural belonging. For Grace, the cloaked stranger was coming to 'take me either … [she pointed up] or [she pointed down]'.

The humorous story is something of a 'reconstructive activity', easily recognized in children's play. 'When reality does not fit in with the child's wishes, s/he assigns the desirable traits to an undesirable reality: in the absence of toys the stone becomes a car. The child knows that the stone is a stone but the quality of life is enhanced if it becomes a car for a while' (Salander *et al.* 1996: 992). Similarly, when unpalatable facts are couched by an entertaining narrative, a horror story can seem a joke. It is not necessary to brutally 'literalize' meanings to the narrator, but to enter their reality as it is presented, that is, to accept the laughter, but to hear the tears. 'It is very much a question of being sensitive to the patient's reconstructed reality. Using the image of the playing child, we find a parallel in the parent's sensitivity to the play and to the meaning of the toys. A stone is a car and not a boat! Destroying the child's illusion may result in despair' (Salander *et al.* 1996: 994).

Language of spirit: symbolic form

The second distinguishing aspect of a language of spirit is its exploitation of symbolic form. At this point, a brief 'refresher' on some of the features of symbol seems appropriate. The symbol participates in that to which it points, but its potential for numerous interpretations makes it impossible to 'literally' translate its meaning. In this sense, the symbol transcends its own medium. It may 'show' or imply, but it does not 'say'. All facets of human experience may be embraced by symbol and by holding together apparently contradictory features, fresh meaning is sometimes disclosed. Thus, symbol may mediate something of infinity through the finite or of ultimate meaning via the near at hand, making it possible for us to appreciate multiple levels or dimensions of reality. Apprehension of a symbol sometimes carries profound ontological implications, captivating the observer to such a degree that even the intolerable may begin to seem bearable.

Features of a language of spirit, considered here in terms of symbolic form, include the implicit but nevertheless powerful themes that sometimes permeate discourse, certain selective symbolic meanings and 'motifs of spirit', potentially ritualized behaviour and the various functions of silence. All are traceable in patient narrative and behaviour.

Permeating themes: hearing 'then' in 'now'

Sometimes it is helpful to identify the era wherein words more genuinely resound. When it is suspected that a parent or a teacher can be heard more clearly than the person actually speaking, deep vulnerabilities may be exposed or, conversely, an inner source of strength. As a Catholic child, Judith went to a convent school: 'It was very fear oriented—do this or that or you'll go to hell. I know I could have done better. I used to yell at the kids, I could have had a better career. Of course. It's all too late now. There are lots of things I would have liked to have changed.' Although unspoken, one suspects the final line of many school reports resonates through this self-deprecation: 'Judith could do better if she tried'. Beyond that, perhaps the distant rumblings of the *Ars moriendi* literature of the late middle ages where dying well is like cramming for an examination and it is one's state during the last moments that counts eternally. Certainly, Judith regarded her own dying as an enormous test; 'it's sort of like an exam that you've got to take. In my youth you had to take them, no matter what. You couldn't escape. You could only hope that what you had learned would come up. Dying is like that, whatever good you've done, hopefully, comes up more than the evil. I just hope I haven't been that wicked.'

Listening for the 'unspoken echo' in an utterance is not without danger, but it may suggest potential sources of comfort. A sensitive, explicitly theological conversation may have relieved some of Judith's 'pre-finals anxiety'. She enjoyed discussing her religion with the hospice chaplain and such an approach would merely have followed where Judith herself was leading: 'My religion helps me up to a point … but now … [softly, almost whispering] it isn't working very well now …'. Disarming the metaphor of judgement, from within a supportive theological discourse, would simultaneously have respected Judith's views, honoured her heritage and reinforced her sense of 'belonging' to a community of faith, so protecting an already vulnerable woman from accusations of childish logic. Relaxing the stranglehold of this metaphor over Judith's world view may have rendered more compassionate and optimistic possibilities. In this instance, religious and spiritual needs coincide.

It is not uncommon for the implicit content of speech to reveal as much, or more, than its explicit counterpart. Images of illness, for example, imply what it means to be healthy. To have cancer is to be 'shattered' (Victor), 'broken up, in bits and pieces' (Sadie) or 'all disintegrated' (Carla). Although many people half anticipated their diagnosis of cancer, for a sizeable number, its receipt was recounted in violent terms such as: 'My blood [results] was all up the wall', 'I was knocked back' or 'It was a blow, a hit'. Persistent malevolence and stealth anthropomorphize cancer: 'I don't trust it, it's a nasty disease' (Mary); 'The thing's not gone—it just won't go away' (Elsie); 'It burrowed its way up through me skin to the bottom of me spine to get out. No wonder I was in pain' (Edwin); 'It's gonna poke its ugly head up again' (Sadie). Tracey's description of a negative itinerant force is particularly chilling, 'It's an alien inside my body. It takes over and eats you. It's a monster eating me away, a dark grey-black colour. It shoots from one person to another. It doesn't die with you, it's a living thing that eats you dry and then moves on.'

This is 'magical thinking' (Rozin et al. 1986) at its most powerful, where a plea for exorcism, comparable with any of the middle ages, articulates the desire for health, for health is the antithesis of such possession and is synonymous with integrity and wholeness. To be well is to be free, to belong to oneself and to regard one's body with affection. Such aspirations form the core values of modern palliative care and, relying upon a dimensional rather than compartmentalized view of human experience, they support the assertion that good palliative care is also good spiritual care. Influencing one dimension—be it physical, psychological, social or spiritual—inevitably influences all others because they interpenetrate and are mutually constitutive. Considered in this light, Merton's observation that 'everywhere we find at least a natural striving for interior unity and intuitive communion with the Absolute' (Bailey 1987: 193) is hardly surprising, even if usually expressed in more prosaic terms: 'There must be something wider and bigger. I can't believe we're the only ones in the universe, it would be too lonely' (Sadie); 'There must be something after death, it doesn't just stop. There must be something out there' (Tracey).

The notion of the 'absent presence', whether the echoing schoolteacher's reprimand or implicit notions of health, serves to remind, yet again, of the informing tension that exists in any symbol system. Eunice provides a particularly interesting example of the 'invisible' shaping the apparent. Despite receiving careful explanations of the interviewing procedure, she paused part way through to express some disappointment, 'I imagined there would be a lot of people all with exactly the same complaint. Then you know you are not the only one. If there were people who had the same complaint, you could talk to each other and not be the only one. You feel you're the only one.' She seemed exasperated by my apparent inability to grasp her increasingly personified argument: 'Well, with someone the same as you, you could help each other. See, I could help her and she could say how she felt, and I could say how I felt. You could get together and help each other instead of being by yourself.' Only at the very end of her interview, Eunice casually remarked 'When I was young, I had a twin. She did everything, she spoke for me and done everything. She was the brainy one—and I was half an hour older. She died 3 years ago.' There is a double defiance of the 'natural order' in this story: the younger twin was the more capable yet, despite the birth order, died first. This was the only mention of Eunice's sister but suddenly a number of things fell into place: the repeated emphasis of her single status, the need to share experiences with someone just like herself and the frustrations of being weak, compounded by the 'abandonment' by the all-capable partner. Part of Eunice's distress seemed to lie in the failure of others (such as myself) to 'see' what, to her, was obvious. Although her physical pain appeared well controlled (until admission she had successfully managed in her warden-controlled flat), a lament for the lost twin suffused her interview. Never explicitly stated, yet clearly contributing to her distress, was the knowledge that she could never be returned what might 'really help', someone just like her. From this perspective, Eunice's was a hopeless situation and she took the view 'they shoot a lame horse, but if a human being is on their last legs, they let them suffer. They give them things to help, but it doesn't really.'

Eunice seems to typify many older people struggling under the burden of multiple losses and it is interesting to speculate whether, had she been 40 years younger, the loss of her twin would have been flagged up as having potentially devastating emotional consequences. Certainly, scant attention was paid in her notes and nursing care plan to her relatively (in the context of a long life) recent bereavement.

If Eunice's lament lay implicit in nearly all she said, knowledge of Victor's Jewish spiritual and cultural legacy brings a depth of meaning to an apparently simple action: the crating and sending of his carpentry tools to his son. Articulating a traditional Jewish viewpoint, Victor saw little possibility for life after death: 'I don't think there is anything afterwards. You can't have eternal life. There has to be that cycle. No, we are here today and gone tomorrow, there's no way of stopping it.'

Here today, gone tomorrow. The individual dies yet the cycle of life remains. It is the creative potential of this life that is treasured and fostered—building a family, a home and a business. This is man's side of the covenant. Although Victor regarded himself as irreligious, 'My Jewishness is more cultural than religious—we just stick to the dietary laws because they're cleaner', he soon revealed a beneath-the-skin orthodoxy. Passing his carpentry tools to his eldest son is an act as spiritually significant as Isaac's giving of the father's blessing. The responsibility of the covenantal relationship passes to the next generation. To know one is dying with a 'good name', 'in credit', is a tremendous consolation and Victor derived comfort from remembering the achievements of his life: his ascent from the basement tailoring business of his father to a good clerical post, his happy marriage, his contented family life and the knowledge of never once having been in debt.

Such apparently unremarkable reflections, combined with the giving away of the tools, profoundly encapsulate much Hebraic conventional wisdom concerning man's relation to God and point to appropriate forms of support: listening to the sorrow of leaving this life whilst drawing attention to its accomplishments. Such care does not have to be laboured; simply encouraging and admiring a display of photographs of children and grandchildren may reassure.

Given that the most pedestrian action is also a gesture, deep truths may be conveyed by the apparently unremarkable. One of the hospice doctors, for example, once explained how she felt she and her own mother never openly spoke of her mother's dying, 'except for one time, but anyone overhearing would never have guessed'. To manoeuvre her mother's wheelchair it was necessary to move her garden fence to take in some of her neighbour's garden. 'One day, Mum just asked me to make sure the fence was put back. That's when we both knew she wouldn't get better.' Once spiritual needs are understood in dimensional rather than compartmentalized terms, spiritual care may come in many forms. In the words of the Vietnamese Buddhist Hanh, 'when the ultimate touches the ocean it becomes a fish'. The challenge for carers is to recognize this other yet same dimension, to understand that a garden fence may tell us where a woman feels she stands in relation to her death—the ultimate unknowing.

Symbolic meanings and motifs of spirit

In most spiritual traditions the lament is an ancient narrative form, typically an expression of woe and an appeal for explanation: 'You do say "Why? What have I done to deserve this?"' (Elsie); 'I mean you do wonder "Why Me?" But it is you, so hard luck and make the best of it' (Mary). Characteristic of the language of suffering (Soelle 1975), the lament is stylistically 'psalmic' where more of form equates with more of content (Lakoff and Johnson 1980: 172). Fading to a whisper, for example, Elsie's comment 'My circle of friends is going … going … going, either moved or passed away' intones as much as states her social fragility. For others, their story was rhythmically exaggerated or delivered in monotone as they reiterated, yet again, the history of their illness. Clearly, people were unused to telling their story simply for its own sake rather than as a means to an end—a necessary résumé for each new professional. Sometimes, a brevity verging on shorthand was used: 'Well, abridged. I had a bad accident at work. Injured me back. Laid off. Go home. Take pills. Lay down. Wasn't getting any better. See a specialist. [sigh] Following week the wife said we had the keys to a new flat. I told her we had the keys to a new tumour' (Fred).

The key carries symbolic implications of freedom (the new flat), but also of incarceration (the new tumour) and the narrative style loosened only after its introduction, when Fred's sigh acknowledges that events possess dimensions of depth and meaning, as well as of sequence. Once such dimensions are acknowledged, the freedom and space for their sensitive consideration is opened. At this point, carers are presented with a choice regarding whether they wish to understand the reality experienced by their patients, or to remain at the sequential or 'surface' level. It is hard to see how carers can enter these other dimensions without some degree of self-reflection, yet our faith in measurement as the only 'true' guarantor of validity has heightened an attitude of 'crude realism'. Consequently, such dialogue often remains unheard or, because we are uncertain how to respond, it is ignored—truly becoming the lament in the wilderness. The nurse dressing the heels of an elderly lady is thus able to ignore her patient's comment 'They're sore because I've been kicking the bucket for too long' and the 'joke' 'I'm heavy enough for 10 men, nine dead and one dying' may be left hanging by those lifting an elderly gentleman up his bed. Each of these events occurred during the period of participant observation although, from the response of staff, it was as if neither comment existed. They landed in a void.

Clearly obdurate examination of every 'throwaway' line is uncalled for, but many 'asides' or illogical comments are cues to deeper needs. It would have been easy to misinterpret or underestimate the seriousness of an allegation made by 38-year-old James. Despite his contradictory signature, James insisted that the hospice was retaining money he had handed over for safekeeping. At best, his adamance was unreasonable, at worst, antagonistic. It is easy for hard-pressed carers to allow such anger to heighten their own resistances, forgetting that to be 'short changed'—of years of marriage, of seeing two small children grow up, of a successful career—could feel like having been cheated or robbed and that anger is a natural passionate lament. Similarly, why should a man waking at 04:40 hours each day, dressing himself and waking his fellow patients in the process, persistently ask his nurses to weigh him? Did the request for scales, ancient symbol of justice and reckoning, express deep fears? His own account of his insomnia might suggest so, 'Well, everything is *in the balance* now ... sleeping is a bad sign; anything can happen when you are asleep.'

This 'symbolic discourse' is emphasized, not simply for its intrinsic interest, but to convince carers of the need to value such communication. Through a heightened awareness of symbols, precious insights to otherwise silent needs may be gleaned. Their expression ought not to be frustrated for they 'address the psyche on different levels, through modes of understanding [other] than the logical ones ... answering the fundamental need to be creative' (Connell 1992:19).

Simon was an ex-municipal gardener in his fifties who lived with his mother. He was a person of acute artistic sensibilities and ability whose favourite activity had been exploring the London art galleries. Opening a box of crayons, one day, his face lit up. Although grey, clammy, unshaven, unable to rise from his chair and worried lest his painful knees be touched, the urgency of his intention and rapid execution was remarkable. As a man possessed, occasionally whistling through clenched teeth and shaking his head, Simon sketched. Thirty minutes later, a magnificent racehorse filled the sheet: chestnut brown, mane flying, galloping from east to west. The jockey leaned forward, urging his mount, which bore the number eight. Clearly satisfied but perspiring heavily and exhausted, Simon announced to no one in particular 'I'm not useless. There's still some hope. Thank God I was made redundant 10 years ago. It was never proper gardening, all that bonus work. I say to you, what's the point in racing each other like that? It's all gone tomorrow and it don't mean a thing then. At least I had them 10 years, thank God, before I'm dying.'

The most precious years of Simon's life defy conventional expectation for he was unemployed. The contrived productivity of bonus-pay gardening was unchallenged, until he realized he was dying. Simon's reverie contains a profound spiritual insight concerning the nature of time and the nature of the 'really real'. All that is physical, even the most potent stallion, is finite. No jockey (degree of consciousness perhaps?) may outrace the setting of the sun. Once this is realized, there is an inversion of priorities: co-operation becomes more important than competition and time 'squandered' in art galleries is the more treasured aspect of a life. The 'real' gardener allows events to unfold according to their nature. There is no manipulation or striving for he works in harmony with time, not against it. For the 'real' gardener a dimension of time is available that is obscured to the labourer shackled to a metaphor of time as a unit of productivity. For him, 'time is money' not an opportunity to 'stand and stare' (Davies, in Albery 1994: 118).

Some clue to the dimension realized by the authentic gardener lies in the number eight on the horse's saddlecloth. A few weeks after Simon died, a senior art therapist working elsewhere was showing me some patients' work when, astonishingly, there appeared a virtually identical painting by a different man. Again, the horse bore the number eight. I was informed that this number frequently appears in the work of terminally ill people, commonly regarded as symbol for infinity because it has no beginning and no end and may be traced in perpetual motion.

In the spiritual writings of most traditions there is a reluctance to dissociate wisdom from some awareness of the ultimate or infinite. It is hard to know whether Simon's painting and commentary point to a profound realization of this truth or indicate a deep yearning for some help to reconcile thoughts on that which carries everlasting value (unlike bonus work)—with the knowledge of his own impending death. St Augustine writes 'Our heart is restless Lord until it rests in thee' (*Confessions* Chapter 1, Verse 1). Put more contemporarily, 'eternity becomes an "experience", the absence of which is not simply a limit that is thought, but a lack that is felt at the heart of temporal existence. This "permeation" with negativity compels lamentation at the way in which the soul deprived of the stillness of the eternal present, is torn asunder' (Clark 1990: 166).

Regardless of whether it is expressed in wax crayon, to contemplate any conciliation of finite and infinite fosters hope insofar as it suggests possibility in the dying person's perception of their reality. Simon discovered and found the strength to say he was not useless through his painting. He marvelled at the depth of his reflection and cherished his creativity, keeping a box of crayons in his room. Carol, who held her brush between her teeth, also suggests that such contemplation does not necessarily have to be expressed in the languages of philosophy, theology or psychology to be healing: 'I learn things about myself from my painting that I didn't know I knew. I am totally taken over. It's always enjoyable.' Philosophical and other discourse, after all, are languages of a second order, the experiences she describes comes first.

Simon's 'I say to you [what's the point in racing each other like that?]' recalls the archaic and biblical 'I say unto you' and apparently serves a similar purpose, adding gravitas to his observations and emphasizing their authenticity. Mayo (1996: 211) also comments upon the disclosive potential of archaic language when it arises in vernacular discourse. Just such a juxtaposition occurs in Julia's recollection of a dream that followed or accompanied (she was unsure which) a cardiac arrest. She was 'sitting on a hillside with a wonderful landscape in front of me, trees and mountains and greenery. All the kingdoms of the world were spread out in front of me. It was mine, mine for the taking. In the Bible, temptation is usually a bad thing, whereas this was really positive.'

For Mayo, the ascent, the archaic 'kingdoms', the mountain top vista with its associations of gift or temptation possess powers of disclosure only at a psychological level, but this is also the language of a theological realism, something acknowledged by Julia herself: 'I'm not a Christian but I do believe very strongly in a creator. Suddenly everything seemed very simple, like God's name: I AM. God is, and everything is just so simple … it's almost impossible to describe, but the universe is so orderly. All we have to do is to get ourselves into that order. I don't want to get into theological discussions and my Catholic background does tend to show, but suddenly I was conscious that all I had to do was to get myself as ordered and I would be healthy and correct, correct in the sense of that's how I am supposed to be. It sounds crazy if I say it, but it's as if God was the bones of the universe.'

The ultimate as supporting structure of the universe: it is hard to think of a better description of the *anima mundi* (McFague 1993). Julia's Catholic background shows only because it provides her with at least some rudimentary vocabulary for what she finds so difficult to say about human encounters with ultimate 'landscapes'. Despite her protests, her contemplation of her dream is a theological exercise and her need to speak of it expresses a yearning for theological discourse. A discourse not necessarily couched in conventional religious terminology but ideally conducted with someone able to detect the ancient motif of the *anima mundi* and to appreciate its contemporary implication. There is a connection between the idea of the soul of the world and the notion of enchantment where 'every single object of nature and culture [is] alive with personality and subjectivity' (Moore 1996: 187) that resonates with Julia's return to consciousness after her medical crisis. Everything is the same but seen in a new, almost iridescent way: 'the next morning, a nursing assistant was singing at the next bed as she made it. She had a beautiful voice. All of a sudden, my hearing came back full force. It was the sweetest thing I had ever heard. My sister brought me some delphiniums, a really glowing blue. So blue, so bright, almost burning, you could almost see the colour burning away in the air. Each sense seemed to come back one at a time and I felt so peaceful and full of understanding of how things were. Somebody died that night and there was this sense of peacefulness over it. It certainly helped me get through the first few days. Then, of course, ordinary daily life starts to impinge again.'

Human understanding of the ultimate is conventionally presented in masculine terms whereas the *anima mundi* presents a feminine face. Far from being 'crazy', Julia's 'vision' suggests a need to connect with the wisdom of the feminine, something she herself articulated. 'I've used that sort of vision of the order of the universe to imagine my cells as orderly. I used to visualize burning them out. Now I say, "come in to order please. I want you. I want you healthy". Much more gentle. I've gone along with it, but I feel a great dislike for radiotherapy. It's blunt instrument stuff. It's male type medicine. It's back to "burn it out".'

Appropriate spiritual care might have been directed towards a positive acknowledgement and development of Julia's feminine consciousness, possibly in the light of some discussion of the *anima mundi*. The archetypal hero (to be discussed in Chapter 10) was an extremely powerful metaphor for Julia, but it did not always work to her advantage. Despite a certain openness to what Hillman (1977) calls 'imaginal' insights, 'I think that dreams can tell you things about yourself that you just can't arrive at on your own' (Julia), she sometimes seemed very out of touch with her own needs. There were signs, however, that restricting exploration to psychological or physical terrain may have been inappropriate: 'Doctors are supposed to heal and if they can't heal they should offer something active like meditation, but every time I speak to the homecare team it's do I need counselling? But I don't think I need counselling.'

Any unsatisfactory encounter with a patient should challenge carers to unearth the values their practice embodies. When a patient invokes an organizing principle as comprehensive as the *anima mundi,* no less is demanded. Julia's 'vision' encapsulates a world view whereby she wanted to consider her relationships. She and contemporary materialism were out of step: 'My brother lent me a television but I couldn't bear it, the noise, the crudity, the nation has been hit all over with Tory values: gimme, gimme, gimme.' Perhaps the repeated offers of counselling were frustrating because her 'problems' were signs, not of pathology, but of awareness and growth. Very often, other needs do not surface until physical pain is dealt with, but 'every time the homecare team came to see me, or telephoned, they just asked me if I was in pain, but I don't think pain is necessarily to be got rid of. I'd rather have some pain and be alert.'

For Julia, her physical needs were met. A more sensitive response may have been some form of spiritual 'direction'/exploration couched in an acceptable terminology. Julia realized that an explicitly 'religious' response would have been unhelpful: 'I don't think services will do'. A positive evaluation of her feminine consciousness and an introduction to writing on the *anima mundi*, combined with a course of meditation or gentle yoga may have been more helpful to this highly articulate and sometimes intimidating woman than repeated offers of analgesia and counselling.

If a direct association with the *anima mundi* exists in Julia's dream, Carla's interview brings to mind the ancient spiritual motif of the mandala. This Hindu word originally meant magic circle. Although never directly mentioned, its invocation is permissible from the perspective of the linguistic structuralist, for whom, in addition to its content, the underlying structure of language carries meaning. This meaning is disclosed, not by direct observation, but by inference from data. When these principles are applied to Carla's interview transcript it is hard to avoid the presence of the mandala. Featuring in Tibetan, Eastern and Indian art, the dances of the Navaho native people, the Rose windows of cathedrals and contemporary architecture, the mandala has an ancient and diverse heritage signifying the relation of the cosmos to divine powers (Jung 1964: 266–85).

Traditionally comprising a series of concentric rings intersecting with a quadrilateral form, the mandala assists the observer to enter a meditative state where meaning and order in life is apprehended and a feeling of deep peace is experienced. In Jungian terms, roundness symbolizes a natural wholeness or psychic completion and the quadrangular formation indicates its realization in consciousness. Carla, feeling marginal to family life and physically restricted, however, speaks only of circles, creating a powerful sense of enclosure and frustration: 'I'm on the edge of the family circle now. I want to do something about it. I want to be at home but I've moved to the edge. I started to watch a cookery programme this evening and I really wanted to go home to cook them a big meal and I couldn't.' For Carla, the very ordinariness of the cookery programme is a poignant reminder of how far she has moved from the heart of her family. For her, the dining table—conventional icon of family unity—speaks not of communion but exclusion.

The contradiction between circle and quadrilateral in the mandala is a visual representation of the insoluble problem: squaring the circle—a preoccupation of alchemists and the ancient Greeks. For Carla, trapped in her room, the mandalic structure is appropriately frustrating: 'I can only stand on one leg for a couple of moments. My range of movement is only an arm's length [gesticulating], a circle. I can't move other than in a small circle.' Moreover, regardless of her efforts, Carla knew that her situation was fundamentally unalterable: 'While I was having the operation, then traction, I forgot about the cancer but now my hip is recovering, I've come full circle. I'm fighting the cancer again, back where I started … but, if you want to face it, there is no way it can get better.'

When asked if anything was with her in her circle, she responded 'Trying to make the best of it. Trying to work out why, when I'm so young, I'm only 49.' Here is a problem insoluble to logic, although approachable via meditative contemplation. There is, however, yet a third circle, a private inner life, nestled deep within the concentric patterns of the 'arm's reach' on the perimeter of family life. 'Everything is going on around me, and here I am, in my little circle, with my thoughts and my little life inside my head. Not many people know about this because not many people talk to me about it deeply like you do, but some days I feel so sure about everything, and the next, I don't know what to think or believe. I'm all in a mess.'

In the Islamic tradition especially, this is the type of 'mess' that contemplation of the mandala, by bringing a sense of order and meaning, transforms into creative possibility. Paradoxically, immediately after the exposure of her inner, normally hidden confusions, Carla invoked the primary spiritual functions of the mandala—achievement of a comfort inexplicable to logic, connection with a larger reality and personal transformation, here symbolized by new clothes in a colour traditionally associated with cosmic awareness and tranquillity: 'I find it helpful going to communion. I feel close to God, but I don't understand. I know Jesus Christ was a good man. He died on the cross, and all that, but I don't know if he was the Son of God. I'm not sure. My husband's been seeing a psychotherapist to help him cope and he's going to learn to meditate. I wish I could learn to do something like that. I have a relaxation tape and in the end you see yourself all in a blue dress in a blue light and it is so beautiful. I feel so warm and peaceful.'

Although highly artistic, Carla based many of her paintings on printed illustrations of famous works. She may have found copying an existing mandala in the presence of a sensitive listening companion deeply therapeutic. This could have been presented as a contemplative as well as an artistic pursuit and so satisfied her desire to meditate. Perhaps other patients or staff could have joined her in this activity, so overcoming some of her feelings of exclusion and isolation. Carla was particularly anguished over the issue of whether she should receive communion in the Anglican Church when she was unsure of its significance. My opinion was solicited. I felt that a 'non-response', a deferment to 'interviewer impartiality' or a knee-jerk referral to the hospice chaplain would have betrayed the intimacy of Carla's own disclosures, so I replied, perhaps somewhat feebly, 'Christ invited people to take and eat, not to take and understand'. Although this seemed favourably received, I suspected that Carla's deeper need was not for an answer, but for the security to abandon her logical approach in favour of an intuitive, trusting, 'heartfelt' response. The meditative exercises she craved, whether based on the mandala (Dahlke 1992) or some other technique, may have made this possible. Certainly her desire to learn indicates that, at some level, Carla realized such knowledge may not be 'given' by another, only discovered for oneself, for 'the lyricism of meditative thinking goes right to the fundamental without passing through the art of narrating' (Ricoeur, in Clark 1990: 166).

Ritual

Even bizarre or illogical behaviour is comprehensible when considered in terms of ritual. Take, for instance, this behaviour of a friend. Her 12-year-old son died in a freak and tragic accident. For a long time afterwards, however, in a tender domestic expression of love and grief, he was regularly 're-membered' to his family. Whenever my friend put some washing in the machine, she would include one of his shirts and iron it along with everything else. In her words 'At one level, I knew it was a stupid thing to do, but I simply had to. But I also knew that I wouldn't stay like that forever.'

Ritual is essentially a language of demonstration where actions of the body say more than words. Especially helpful when people feel threatened, ritual can provide a security, a sense of being 'held', particularly in transitional or liminal situations. As Ward and Wild remind (1996: 10), 'when our thoughts cannot move us forward ritual often can.' As anyone who has put a fretful child to bed knows, the curtains must be 'just so', the evening drink in just the right place, the stories read in exactly the right order or sleep will be resisted. If they become compulsive, rituals may imprison, but they also contain a liberating potential. Vulnerability becomes tolerable and there is an opportunity to see things anew. At times of illness especially, Ward and Wild note, we yearn for home, for familiarity. The creative 'holding' of ritual can subvert 'strangeness' in ways that bring comfort but are not always immediately recognizable to 'non-participants'. Without understanding its full import, a private ritual such as Arthur's saluting of each man who left his bay for the mortuary, may be dismissed as a personal eccentricity or 'psychologized' in reductive terms. In the following poem, Carol explains why she insisted her curtains were left open each night, revealing what she called 'my beacon, guiding me home.'

Candle in the sky

Rising up from the trees
Across the road from St Christopher's
Is a TV aerial at Crystal Palace.
Functional, directional or just objectionable to some
But to me, it's my candle in the sky.

The top gleams as white
Against a blue sky.
Drawing my attention I cannot avoid its beckoning light.
Sometimes a dark cloud dims
My candle in the sky
I stare at its obscurity
Defy it to hang around.
It works—clouds move away
My beacon's alight, I'm happy again.

How easy it would be to deny Carol, unable either to gesticulate or to speak, this source of spiritual support—for there is little doubt she interpreted the beacon as ultimately significant, by routinely drawing her curtains. This kind if insensitivity would match a whisking away of the dying flowers that helped Hazel to 'let go'. Carol's poem is no mere artefact; the effort required for its production and her intense desire to communicate deny its triviality; 'it's my feelings outpoured. I put all my thoughts in my poems. I have lots waiting to be expressed, so I have a sense of urgency, of time running out.'

Silence

From a non-essentialist position, defining silence is less important than showing its effects and how it works (Jaworski 1993: 29). We can communicate without speaking or speak in order to maintain silence about something else. Language has been described as a cord of silence with words as its knots (Illich 1973). Its skilful acquisition requires us to listen carefully for the meaning of both. Silence is also a cultural variable (Davidhizar and Newman Giger 1994). Consider the scene where, before addressing her class, a teacher pauses for a moment. Later, one child refuses to answer a question, even when directly addressed, another never raises his hand throughout the entire lesson. Where the teacher uses silence to assert her authority and to create a sense of anticipation, the first child's silence perhaps indicates he is angry for being singled out. The second child, however, is an American Navajo, taught from infancy not to highlight the inadequacies of others by appearing to know more. His silence is an expression of modesty and sensitivity.

As this simple example shows, it is easy to analyse silence in terms of duration and frequency but its ambivalent meaning is far harder to interpret. Conventional or formulaic silences may not even be 'heard' when dealing with people from other cultures. 'When your patient is silent' (Davidhizar and Newman Giger 1994) can indicate anything from a mark of respect, a need for 'thinking time', comfort or discomfort, emotional withdrawal, a desire for privacy, anger, anticipation or expectation, agreement or resistance, a sense of camaraderie or exclusion or it may be symptomatic of certain organic problems such as memory loss. Jensen (1973) identifies five functions of silence, assigning positive and negative values to each: linkage—silence may bond or separate people; affecting—silence may heal or wound over time; revelatory—silence may either hide something or make it known; judgemental—silence may indicate either assent or dissent; and finally, an activating function—silence indicates either deep thoughtfulness or mental inactivity.

Silence can also operate as a control, contriving invisibility for minority or oppressed groups. Gunaratnam (Field *et al.* 1997: 184) for instance, argues that the cultural 'fact files' found on many hospice wards are 'inextricably tied up with the bureaucratic need for the management of difference, reflecting organizational rather than user-oriented interests. Moreover, by staying silent about racism they also serve to negate the influence of structural and inter personal power relations. Far from being innocuous, this silence can actively 'speak' about the legitimate limits of multi-cultural competencies.'

Various metaphors indicate the potential of silence to influence, 'her silence helped him to make up his mind', or suggest that 'silence is a substance', we speak of a 'wall' or 'blanket' of silence. Envisaging silence as a substance we attribute to it various characteristics. 'Silence can be long, heavy, cold or hard' (Jaworski 1993: 82–3). There is a further ontological metaphor: 'silence as container'. For instance, 'the nurse washed him in silence' or 'they touched in silence'. Considered in spatial terms, silence becomes a place where different events may occur—much as the different rooms in a house have different functions.

Silence has come to be seen as something at our disposal. It is often discussed in terms of techne, of a skill to be mastered, over those of poiesis, a mode for unpredictable and novel disclosures. When it is not oppressive, silence may be an excellent technique to encourage communication, but the notion that we use silence is being fostered at the expense of a wider picture. Manuals of communication rarely suggest that, somehow, silence may 'use' or change us or that silence can operate as a symbol or create a space for other powerful symbols to emerge and for something new to happen. Countless individuals from many cultures and traditions have entrusted themselves to silence in the hope of spiritual growth: 'Be still and know that I am God' (Psalm 46). In Zen, truth and silence are inextricably linked so that 'Those who know, do not speak. Those who speak do not know' (Watts 1985: 97). If silence can mediate a transforming encounter, make disclosures of an Ultimate bearing, it is surely part of a vocabulary of spirit and carers should be alert to this possibility (as well as the many others suggested earlier). It may not always be appropriate to regard the silent or withdrawn patient as problematic or depressed.

Silence as paradox

Just as the child who plays with a stone as if it were a toy 'carries' both realities without apparent contradiction, in all spiritual traditions paradox expresses truths via 'non-sense'. Paradox appeals primarily to wisdom rather than to logic, baffling the principle of contradiction whereby a proposition may not be true and false at the same time. Instead of only approaching paradox in terms of irreducible difference, however, it is possible to argue that all experience is analogical in that all human situations carry some of the characterizing 'is/is not' tension of metaphor and that it is from this tension that new meanings emerge. Thus, Tracey may have found the bittersweet quality of Christmas to be insoluble but, in her own words, she was 'well pleased' to be at home: 'I never thought I'd get this far. I'm happy and sad all at the same time.' Similarly, 4 months before her death, Carla remarked 'I can hear two melodies. I do want to give up, but I don't want to. There are things that I actually enjoy, but they are always marred by this' [pointing to her huge abdomen].

Paradox is not about the resolution of a dilemma. Paradox involves cohabiting with diverse aspects of a situation in such a manner that their contradictions are transcended. Taking in her own situation from a different vantage point, even the tensions Carla endured were sometimes bearable: 'I've just got to leave it all in God's hands really, and leave it all with the people who pray for me.' This was said not with a depressed or stoic resignation but intimated a wider horizon against which contemporary events might make some sense— even if Carla herself could not see it.

Tragic humour or contemporary phenomena recounted in archaic terms illustrate how any aspect of a language of spirit may present as a paradox. Silence however, is paradox *par excellence*, 'intensely "there" and, with equal intensity, "not there". The passivity of silence is hard to explain, since in one respect it is intensely active' (Beckett 1995: 24). Accepting this tension enables us to understand meditation as a form of 'silent music' (Johnston 1974); it explains why a man should murder his silent wife so that she says no more (Cox and Theilgaard 1987: 116) and why an 'exemplary' nurse can claim 'the most powerful words in the human language may be those that are never said' (Perry 1996: 9).

Approaching silence in this way is humbling for, like all metaphoric or symbolic disclosures, it resists any total explanation. Robinson (1974) also argues that silence can be a period of gestation, slowly exploring or 'sifting' us so that the essential in a given situation emerges. We may find that, hitherto, we were living as a stranger both to ourselves and to life's deeper meaning. With this knowledge may come a sense of liberation, of direction or even of frustration because others cannot see what, for us, has become obvious. Seer, stranger, silence as a refuge or a challenge, each of these points anticipates the detailed and illustrated discussions of the following chapters.

Silence, as Eastern spiritual traditions acknowledge in their emphasis on posture, breathing, meditation, 'letting go' and emptiness, is not simply an external matter but involves a shifting of attention. So understood, silence can signify inner qualities. Its practitioner may sense a 'coming home' to one's true (in the sense of most complete) nature. In all traditions this includes a spiritual or ultimate dimension. Through disciplined silence and an attitude of availability rather than of attempted control, the individual is consciously attempting to realize their potential as symbol and it becomes difficult to resist the metaphor 'depths of silence'. The notion that the functionally transparent or the culturally conditioned silence may operate symbolically and so lead to personal transformation may, for some, veer too close to notions of an absolute silence. Inherently essentialist, such a stance cannot be maintained for sceptics. After all, if absolute silence exists, does absolute speech? Such a question, however, betrays an understanding of speech and silence more in terms of definitive mutual exclusion than in terms of the is/is not tension of symbol and paradox, thereby depriving silence of its mystery.

Just as there exists an intensity where light is no longer light, in that it does not illuminate but blinds, it is interesting to speculate whether, in defiance of 'common sense', silence has the potential to deafen. Just as Oedipus plucked out his own eyes and then ranted against the dark, spiritual practitioners of all traditions warn of the internal cacophony encountered in silence. When silence is approached only in a positivist way, however, as a discrete component of discourse, frame or some other analytical process, is there not a sense in which it is betrayed? Unless apprehended as symbol, silence is disallowed from speaking its own solution—that which relativizes the tensions of any 'is/is not' situation. These are times when silence 'answers' the logically insoluble, so finding itself allied with wisdom: 'Contradictions have always existed in the soul of man. But it is only when we prefer analysis to silence that they become an insoluble problem. We are not meant to resolve all contradictions but to live with them and rise above them and see them in the light of exterior and objective values that make them trivial by comparison' (Merton 1993: 82).

There is, of course, a certain irony in speaking or writing about silence. Against those who find much of what has been said here to be obtuse or abstract, this notion of silence as symbol is offered in the spirit of an invitation not a 'final word'. Knowledge about silence does not substitute for experience thereof. Furthermore, our primary concern remains the experiences of patients. To this end, the following account of Claire's interview is offered, both as the motivation for this discussion and as illustration of its argument: that silence sometimes loosens the stranglehold of conventional expectations and this can allow novel insights or symbolic disclosures to emerge and that these disclosures are occasionally so healing that, in theological terms, they may be described as graced, their implications extending beyond psychological or emotional parameters.

Claire's nurses had suggested that the evening might be the best time for me to meet her, as she liked to rest in the afternoon. When I entered her side room, the light was dim and Claire lay on her bed. Single and in her early forties, Claire once held a responsible City position, as well as caring for her elderly parents. Later, she spoke wistfully of her Russell and Bromley handbags, expensive shoes and of dining at Frederick's. Although her fingernails were beautifully manicured and polished, her hair was unkempt and she was slumped to one side. Her unflattering tracksuit was grubby and a full catheter bag protruded from one trouser leg.

Within moments of my entering, Claire began to sob. Enormous tears rolled down her cheeks, her eyes closed, her nose ran: 'It's because I'm not in charge of my body any more. I need to get this stuff [that is, phlegm] off my chest but I can't roll over. I've got lung cancer and I'm so pissed off. I never smoked in my life. The whole problem is, my father's very ill. [barely audible] … I think he looks at me and keeps saying "Why, why did I have to have a daughter like that?" But I spent all my time running up and down the King's Road in Chelsea getting things for him. I think even our doctor might have said "You've done this to her." I feel so angry … like the devil. [even more softly] But I was going to be the one to look after them …'

Claire closed her eyes and lay back against her pillows. The atmosphere in the room felt charged and I was reluctant to break the silence. After a few moments, without any warning, Claire began to shout with real aggression in her voice: 'This … all this … it's made me realize what a disgusting scam the national lottery is; they give all those thousands of pounds to African tribal dances … I JUST DON'T THINK THAT YOU SHOULD GIVE MONEY TO PEOPLE TO DANCE AROUND LIKE THAT … IT ISN'T FAIR …'

As she shouted, Claire also sobbed and large gobbets of green sputum covered her hands. She lay back again, clearly exhausted and repulsed. Fetching a cloth and some water, with her permission, I gently and slowly washed and dried her hands. The washing assumed a dignity I had never before experienced as a nurse and the silence was interrupted only once by Claire murmuring 'something is coming to a natural ending here'. The evening light was fading so I turned on another lamp. Any tension had dissolved and the room felt calm. Claire thanked me for listening to her. We sat quietly together for a little while then chatted about the inconsequential: clothes, nail varnish, women's magazines. I arranged to return later in the week. Her rapid deterioration, however, prevented this and Claire died two days afterwards.

There is something in this story that resonates with the experiences of long-suffering Job. His comfort arrives when he 'receives an answer from God. But what God says to him does not answer the charge, it does not even touch upon it. The true answer Job receives is God's appearance only, only this, that distance turns into nearness that his eyes "see him". Nothing is explained, nothing adjusted; wrong had not become right, nor cruelty kindness' (Robinson 1974: 14). Similarly, nothing in this incident with Claire altered the unfairness of her situation. There were no ready answers to remedy her anger. Even so, there is little doubt that she found her 'interview' extremely comforting and, perhaps unsurprisingly, there was a quality of ritual, an excess of meaning, in the hand washing, for 'water symbolizes the whole of potentiality: it is the *fons et origo*, the source of all possible experience ... water symbolizes the primal substance from which all forms come and to which they will return' (Eliade 1979: 188).

If any further comments are required, they concern notions of timing and silence. There are occasions when it is appropriate to trust silence to provide or prompt the appropriate response. Like a good idea, the right word or the ideal symbolic gesture is not of our own making, but a 'given' that favours (sometimes) earlier preparation. The deepest disclosures are never forced. Although purely fortuitous, Claire's interview seemed neither a moment too soon, nor a moment too late. Had she told her story, 'broken her silence', only the week before, perhaps our encounter would have been more 'conventional'. Those who find such reflections hyperbole are a valuable counterbalance to the dangers of sentimentalism and projection (hence the value of team work). They too, however, must be familiar with the experience of not wishing to 'break' a silence, the instinctive recognition that the 'right moment' has not arrived.

Western society, however, generally treats speech as normal and silence as deviant. It is more 'normal' for silence to be unwelcome or discomforting. For many, however, advancing illness is something of a movement into silence, a gradual withdrawal from the cut and parry of their conventional 'language games'. When silence comes unbidden through sensory loss, social isolation or the refusal of others to communicate frankly, individuals can experience painful and dislocating sensations of estrangement. The practice of silence may be simple, but rarely is it easy. The ingenious efforts of some patients to restructure temporal metaphor is perhaps as much a bid to 'drown' the discomforting effects of silence though activity as an attempt to regain control over their situation (see Chapter 6).

The 'is/is not' of silence is, however, a totality. Even when transposed to a visual medium, as in the 'spaces' of a sculpture or the 'emptiness' of a Japanese garden, silence can be powerfully eloquent. If the important 'silent half' of a story is to emerge, however, courage may be required, for silence can be painful. Jaworski (1993: 151) draws attention to the American artist Edward Hopper whose work is characterized by the power of the unspoken. He poses the question of silence as a discomforting absent presence. For example, how does a room look when no one is there to see it? This speculation may strike as somewhat abstract but it often resonates through patients' commonly expressed concerns. As Eileen puts it, 'the trouble is, I want to make my will, but I want to be here to see it fulfilled.' Again resonating with forthcoming discussions, many of Hopper's subjects are placed in liminal or transitional locations: windows, doorsteps, verandas and balconies.

If silence repels it can also, sometimes simultaneously, attract. Many patients noted with appreciation the peace and quiet of St Christopher's. More than once, deliberately constructed quiet times were mentioned: Carla as she painted; Carol staring at her beacon; Fred and Hazel both meditated; Debbie regularly conducted a silent evening recollection of her day. For Eileen, the total containment she seemed to experience in the hospice chapel was comforting: 'I'm calm there. Everything is good.' If patients find themselves caught up in the 'repellent attractiveness' of silence, one can only wonder how they might be helped, if those who listen to them deny silence its symbolic potential—if they fail to recognize silence as part of a language of spirit.

Résumé

In this chapter I have tried to show that interpretations of human spirituality ought not to begin at the level of abstract assertions such as 'God exists', for these are second-order propositions. In searching for a non-religious language of spirit, therefore, I have given priority to the words and actions of patients. From these, it is possible to speak meaningfully of a vocabulary of 'happenings' whose interrelations form a language or network of different 'tools' for expressing ultimate concerns. The relationship between these 'tools' and the language itself has been handled in terms of a gestalt between part and whole. Although fluid and ingenious, this language of spirit has three identifiable aspects: its context, its literary form and its symbolic form. Respective examples include selective vignettes and biographical details, archaic language and humour and permeating themes, symbolic meanings and motifs of spirit, ritualized behaviour and the use of silence. Paradox as a phenomenon that may be found in any aspect has also been considered. Perhaps addressing this language from a slightly different perspective or level, the implications of linguistic structure briefly enter considerations of the spiritual motif of the mandala.

Appendix: participant profiles

Arthur

Arthur was an 83-year-old retired tea blender who spent his days reading his dictionary. Despite the rectorial air this bestowed, he was an avowed sceptic. Stepfather to five children, whose mother had died 9 years previously, Arthur was closest to one particular stepdaughter who was present during his interview. Admitted for respite care, he was reluctant to leave somewhere he 'felt secure' for an unknown nursing home. A stoic gentleman, 'I know what I've got to do, I'll just get on with it', who could sometimes appear abrupt.

Bernard

After many years as managing director of his own company, Bernard, an 81-year-old rather 'dapper' widower, still retained many of the mannerisms of a man at ease when exercising authority. At times, however, he became emotional and embarrassed by what he called his 'stupid' bouts of crying. Cancer of the prostate had spread to Bernard's bones but he was more concerned about his son who was dying from skin cancer. Bernard spent his retirement in a hot climate and wondered whether his son's visits and exposure to the sun had triggered his melanoma. His daughter had died some years previously after a period of alcoholism. Bernard had severed all communication with his girlfriend abroad as there 'seemed no alternative'. He felt it might be best for him to 'be out of the way' in an old people's home until he too died.

Camilla

A 50-year-old nurse suffering from motor neurone disease, Camilla's condition was diagnosed 18 months prior to her admission to St Christopher's where she received total care. A single woman, Camilla had been a great traveller and her room was full of photographs taken on her various adventures. Her cat 'Pinky' moved in with her along with some furniture from her flat and her music centre. A popular person with a dry pithy sense of humour, Camilla was clearly cherished by her friends. She expressed a desire to explore some of the teachings of the major religions whilst she was an in-patient. Camilla died 6 months after her admission, and, on the request of the ward staff and others who had cared for her, a memorial service was held at the hospice.

Carla

Carla was an in-patient at St Christopher's for over a year, a length of stay never anticipated when she was admitted at the age of 48. Originally diagnosed with breast cancer, bone cancer was detected 4 years later. Carla regarded herself as 'interested in spiritualism'—although she was married to a Jew. Before becoming ill she worked as a medical secretary. Carla worried about her two teenage sons, one of whom was at university. Numerous discussions took place with Carla, who loved to paint. Her room became something of an artist's studio—a befitting environment for this imaginative slightly bohemian person whose striking aquamarine and purple clothes recalled her 1960s teenage years.

Carol

By the time of her interview Carol had been suffering from motor neurone disease for 2 years. She was almost entirely paralysed and could communicate only through a 'type-easi' machine. As a child, Carol and her sister had narrowly escaped becoming Japanese prisoners of war in Burma, where she witnessed the assassination of her father and uncle. With a few others, 'we walked for our lives' over the mountains to India. A twice-divorced Catholic, 66-year-old Carol experienced her illness as something of a 'second journey', one of self-discovery and awakening, facilitated, in part, by the poems she wrote and her art therapy sessions.

Claire

Prior to, and for some of her illness (lung cancer was initially diagnosed, later spreading to her brain), 42-year-old Claire enjoyed a glamorous job in the city as an insurance underwriter. She spoke poignantly of her fashionable shoes, clothes, handbags and meals at sophisticated restaurants. An only child and a non-smoker, Claire had nursed both her parents through a series of illnesses. It was hard for her not to resent the way her life had turned out and the apparent unfairness of her situation. Claire regarded herself as a Christian and had turned—despite his criminal record—to a faith healer for help. She wondered whether her continuing deterioration was because she was not believing 'hard enough'. She also felt extremely guilty that she would not be able to continue caring for her parents as she would have wished.

Claude

Once an international businessman, Claude and his wife had enjoyed a 'globe-trotting' life. Only recently retired (he was 61 years old) Claude was clearly used to commanding attention and respect. He and his wife had been planning a 'round-the-world trip' when Claude was diagnosed with lung cancer. A life-long heavy smoker, Claude was relentless in blaming himself for 'ruining' his wife's life. She had always begged him not to smoke. A childless couple with few friends because of their itinerant lifestyle, Claude worried about how his wife would cope alone. Whenever he mentioned her name he began to weep. Although he did not regard himself as religious, Claude increasingly welcomed the support of the hospice chaplain as his illness progressed.

Debbie

Thirty-year-old Debbie, recently married and qualified as a social worker, was the mother of a 9-year-old boy from a previous relationship. Part of a large extended black South London/West Indian family she had daily contact with her mother who cared for her son when Debbie became too ill. As her condition deteriorated, Debbie felt the need to distance herself from her husband and, although they were separated at the time of her death, her other relatives were warm and sympathetic towards him. He too was a social worker. Once a self-confessed 'health and exercise freak', Debbie's weight had more than doubled since she became ill. She suffered from an extremely rare condition in adults (a malignant tumour from the Ethnold sinus) which had swollen and distorted her face. She felt this rarity sometimes made her an object of curiosity.

Edwin

Edwin (aged 51) lived with his girlfriend and her son having, many years earlier, lost any contact with his wife and five children. His marriage collapsed after Edwin left the army and found civilian life too difficult to cope with, perhaps because he was dyslexic. He then joined the foreign legion and served in Africa where he was involved in some distressing incidents. On his return to England, Edwin developed an alcohol problem and was involved in some petty crime. Although he presented frequently at his general practitioner's he felt he was never properly examined and that his rectal cancer was inappropriately treated as a case of severe haemorrhoids. Eventually, faecal matter emerged through the skin of Edwin's back and he was rushed to hospital as an emergency admission. Two weeks later, Edwin was a patient at St Christopher's. Although he lived for another 3 months and was able to return home for short periods, during these visits Edwin sought comfort in alcohol. Edwin was a gentle, sensitive and thoughtful person who had experienced periods of intense suffering in his life. At the time of his interview he was wrestling with some profound existential problems.

Eileen

Eileen was a warm and engaging person, popular with her carers. Aged 63, her husband had died from motor neurone disease at St Christopher's 3 years earlier. Now retired, Eileen had held numerous different jobs in her life, including one as a veterinary assistant. She spoke of her own little dog with amused affection. Eileen had a right partial mastectomy and was well until, 5 years later, a total mastectomy was required. Eileen and her husband did not have a family and she was very dependent upon her neighbours for company. Eileen felt she was turning to religion for support more than she might have expected and was surprised to hear herself 'talking out loud to God', especially at night when she said she sometimes felt 'real despair'.

Elsie

After an extremely active life, including driving an ambulance during the blitz, this frail, single, blind, elderly lady of 83 years was struggling with her increasing social isolation. Suffering from bowel cancer, Elsie said she was both angered and frustrated by her altered circumstances. Living alone in a council flat on a South London housing estate, she was the sole survivor of a large family. Apart from her niece, all family contact was finished and her friends were rapidly disappearing as they too died. Once a convinced Sunday school teacher, Elsie was distressed to find her faith inadequate to her circumstances.

Elspeth

Elspeth had survived for 15 years after her original diagnosis of breast cancer. At the age of 58, however, she was suffering from a reoccurrence with metastases in her bones. Her son had recently married but she was extremely worried about her daughter, 'she clings to me, she hasn't any friends of her own.' Having cared for her own father for many years, Elspeth's deepest fear was that history would repeat itself for her daughter. Before her illness made it impossible, Elspeth worked as a secretary, 'for as long as I possibly could'. She regarded herself as an atheist and was described by staff as 'an obsessive worrier'.

Eunice

At 81 years of age, Eunice was the last surviving child of a family of six children, including her identical twin. She lived in sheltered residential accommodation where she was very happy until becoming ill. Suffering from cancer of the anal canal with some vaginal infiltration, Eunice was deeply afraid of her pain returning and repulsed by the physical consequences of her diagnosis.

Although a widow, Eunice had no family of her own. As a young woman she had worked as a care assistant.

Fred

Although only 49 years old, Fred had retired from his senior management position. He was a very 'chirpy' sort of man who always seemed determined to put a brave face on events, despite the spread of prostate cancer to his bones. His interview took place 5 days before his death and his wife was present. Fred was father to two adult children from a previous marriage and was an enthusiastic handyman at home.

Gregory

Suffering from malignant mesothelioma, perhaps because of exposure to asbestosis in his working life, Gregory was also blind. He was a retired naval officer, tall and well groomed with a gentle air. Father to one daughter and grandfather to two children, Gregory desperately missed his wife who was suffering from senile dementia in a nursing home. The oldest of seven children, it had been decided that Gregory would spend some time with each sibling after his respite admission. His own feelings seemed a little ambivalent about this arrangement.

Hazel

Hazel was 83 years of age and suffering from Parkinson's disease. She was a genteel and intellectual woman who married in her fifties. On outliving her husband, in her mid-seventies she travelled to India alone, 'for both of us'. Her husband had been a classical scholar and they had planned to visit Bede Griffith's ashram together. In her youth, Hazel had studied sculpture in Paris and had been involved in some relief work after the war. Now totally dependent and confined to a wheelchair she was unable to propel (she was afraid of an electric chair), Hazel regarded herself as purposefully engaged in her own spiritual development. She tried to dedicate a certain portion of each day to meditation and reading her Bible. This intriguing, sensitive and surprisingly bold thinker, clearly felt vulnerable to the indignities imposed by age and illness.

Irene

The mother of three adult children, Irene, a 62-year-old housewife had decided to refuse all further active treatment for her multiple myeloma. Although supported in her decision by her family, she felt she was 'chickening out'. Irene did not regard herself as belonging to any faith although she felt envious of those who do 'believe something'. Irene was a quiet resigned person with whom I found it difficult to 'connect'.

Jane

Jane was a 46-year-old nurse who had particularly enjoyed working with eld-erly people. Abandoned as a child, Jane had lived in many foster homes prior to her nursing training. She was separated from her husband who had suffered a stroke. He was cared for by their son. For the last 7 years of her life she had lived with a new partner who she felt could not 'look at things'. When she received her diagnosis of motor neurone disease (2 years prior to her inter-views), Jane took a drug overdose. Although her life was saved, she found it 'comforting to know I can end it all if it becomes too much'. This desire to retain control was typical—Jane stayed at home for as long as possible using a variety of electronic and other aids. It also made her diagnosis hard to bear. Jane died at St Christopher's 2 months after a lengthy interview at her home and a number of subsequent conversations during her respite visits.

Josie

An extremely talkative and overweight 43-year-old divorced mother of two teenage children, with a history of chronic depression, Josie is something of a 'deviant' case (although this was not known at the time of her interview), in that her diagnosis of a malignant brain tumour was mistaken. After perma-nently losing her sight and many months of believing her condition to be ter-minal, Josie was eventually discharged from the care of St Christopher's to the guidance of a disability support unit. She continues to live at home with her youngest child, her 18-year-old daughter. Josie regards herself as an atheist. Her own mother died unexpectedly when Josie believed herself to be termi-nally ill. Josie was extremely sad that her mother never learnt of the misdiag-nosis as she had already lost one child in adulthood.

Judith

The mother of four adult children, Judith (54 years old) was a practising Catholic. Until the diagnosis of a cerebral haemangioma was confirmed, she had worked as a secretary. Prior to her death, Judith spent a number of weeks confined to bed in her side room. She had become extremely large and difficult to nurse. Further complications also meant she was unable to eat other than through a tube directly into her stomach. Despite these challenges, her equa-nimity of temperament and interest in others was admired by all who cared for her.

Julia

A 51-year-old divorcee on good terms with her ex-husband and his new wife, Julia had recently embarked on a law degree after many stressful and combative years working as a housing officer in a deprived London borough. Julia became involved with the Bristol Cancer Help Centre when she was first diagnosed with breast cancer. This re-occurred 10 years later and, at the time of her interview, there was also liver involvement. She was an extremely forthright positive person keen to do anything she felt might maximize her chance of survival. Although raised as a Catholic, Julia found organized religion 'unhelpful'. Julia participated in two interviews, one at her elegantly decorated home on a snowy December day. She died somewhat unexpectedly in her sleep shortly afterwards.

Mary

At 43 years of age, Mary was the busy mother of two young children: a daughter of nine and a son of five. She was treated for rectal cancer 4 years prior to the discovery of lung cancer. This diagnosis was made only 3 months before her interview—which took place 3 weeks before her death. Her hugely distended abdomen made breathing extremely difficult for Mary, who was clearly once an attractive woman. Until her children were born, Mary had worked as a secretary. A practising Christian, Mary regarded her faith as extremely important.

Sadie

Sadie was a confident sociable person. Although married and 48 years of age, she was concerned to find herself falling too much [she felt] into the role of her elderly parents' 'little girl'. Sadie's marriage was her third, finally happy, partnership. She was an only child, without children of her own, feeling torn between her husband and her parents. She freely admitted to being terrified of death and 'mortified' by the changes in her body. Diagnosed as suffering from breast cancer a year earlier, Sadie died 4 weeks after her interview—7 months after learning the cancer had spread to her lungs.

Tracey

The mother of five children, 39-year-old Tracey worked as a care assistant until she became ill. Her eldest child was 19 years old with a baby of her own. Her youngest, a son, was 9 years old. Tracey directed all her efforts towards the support and well-being of her children. Clear and articulate, Tracey saw herself holding together a family with a history of strong tensions.

Victor

Seventy-six-year-old Victor, engaging and talkative, was one of 10 children of Jewish parents. The family were Rumanian refugees to the UK following a particularly vicious pogrom. In his youth, Victor worked in his father's tailoring business and later in a kosher restaurant. His wife was diagnosed as having lung cancer in the same week as himself. His only surviving brother, whom Victor admired greatly for having qualified as a doctor, was also suffering from cancer. Victor was admitted to St Christopher's because 'I was neglecting myself, not washing or eating. I was really down.' He spoke fondly of playing bridge and enjoyed the craft activities in the day centre. A dignified father of two adult children and a great grandfather, Victor's manner and bearing spoke of a particular epoch of European history as well as his personal circumstances.

Other patients who are mentioned were not formally interviewed; their contribution stems from the period of participant observation.

Part 3

Nine metaphors waiting to be recognized — how spirituality is mediated in the here and now

Chapter 6

Patients' sources of meaning and sense of self

Introduction

By identifying various 'tools' of a language of spirit, the previous chapter suggested some of the ways whereby people communicate spiritually significant issues when they do not use a specifically religious language. A shift of emphasis is now in order: away from *how* this language of spirit works, to *what* terminally ill people use it say—towards the metaphors that disclose, mediate and structure their reality. Of course, when considering the communication of meaning, any separation of *how* and *what* is suspect and, to some degree, each metaphor is constructed from different aspects of the linguistic matrix laid out in the preceding pages. Nevertheless, when one closely observes and listens to patients, these metaphors are clearly discernable. It seems appropriate to present them in a symbolic form (Fig. 6.1) for a number of reasons. Firstly, any interpretation is itself a system of symbols. Secondly, metaphors and symbols refuse to be encapsulated by definition. In no sense does this book try to provide any 'final word' on the spirituality of dying people but this does not mean it has nothing useful to say. It has already been argued that science, religion and the arts all rely on metaphor for cognitive purchase for, without needing to be definitive, metaphor can refer to and depict aspects of reality that are otherwise inaccessible. It therefore seems an ideal, possibly the only, way of approaching the slippery topic of spirituality. Finally, the symbol addresses the whole person, not just the intellect. When palliative care aims to improve sensitivity towards the dying person at every level, this seems important. Very often it is not 'what we know', but 'how we are' with patients that makes all the difference to their care.

Figure 6.1 presents the metaphors that mediate reality for terminally ill people as a three-dimensional and nine-faceted prism. Each facet embodies one of the metaphors or archetypes by which patients live, so providing different points of access to their sources of meaning and sense of self. The ninth facet, however, is somewhat mysterious. It represents that 'surplus of meaning' in any event that escapes articulation (Ricoeur 1976). Even while following a

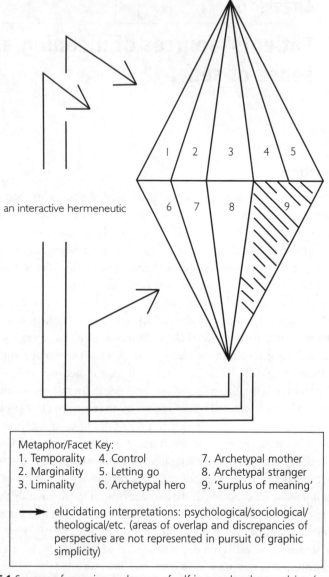

Figure 6.1 Sources of meaning and sense of self in people who are dying (revealed and constructed by metaphor).

necessarily sequential narrative, it is important to remember that the prism is three dimensional. This will help to keep in mind the extent to which its facets influence and inform each other. For example, as it became clear that people mobilize familiar metaphors to cope with the unfamiliar situation of dying, temporal metaphor could be detected in words and deeds that initially seemed unrelated. Similarly, metaphors of control and letting go are mutually implicated and later reflection on the seer is also inadequate without understanding it as 'located' at a cross-sectional point where metaphors of temporality, marginality, liminality and the archetypal stranger 'meet'. Figure 6.1 should be approached holistically for the metaphors it presents are not separate compartments or simply a list of themes or headings.

Approachable from any angle, the prism invites various interpretations: sociological, psychological, anthropological or theological. Each interpretation or hermeneutic is analogous with shining a beam of light at the prism. Inevitably, there are overlaps and discrepancies of perspective, but each discipline claims to have the best or most inclusive view. Inevitably, however, any perspective will also be a distortion and although each discipline legitimately regards its interpretation as total, none is exhaustive. The critical question is which interpretation penetrates furthest, illuminates most brightly and discloses hitherto unseen aspects of reality? In short, which interpretations are the most enticing and make most sense? Certain paradoxes arise here. Consciousness is always consciousness of something. What we know influences what we see, and what we see influences our knowledge. Recalling earlier comments on the hermeneutic circle, therefore, prism and beam are not entirely separate, but interacting. Discovery is about learning to see the already-present in a new way although, paradoxically, this already-present will not be 'there' for us until we see it. A good theory is less about providing new 'facts' than evoking a recognition that shows us the world afresh. Hence the ambition of this book is relatively simple: to draw attention to aspects of patient experience that are currently unrecognized as potential expressions of patient spirituality or spiritual need. It does this by outlining a language of spirit and by exploring various metaphors constructed from this language. Not only do patients use these metaphors to give account of what they experience, the metaphors actually shape and mediate their experiences. The first metaphor to be considered is that of temporality. The remaining eight are those of marginality, liminality, control and letting go, or relate to the archetypal figures of hero, mother and stranger and the final metaphor, of course, deals with life's 'surplus of meaning'.

Metaphors of temporality

If human spirituality is concerned with the quest for meaning, then it is inseparable from our understanding of time. We all need a meaningful temporal framework. The stories we tell about ourselves and why we are here give time its human face. As Sara's poem about her various haircuts demonstrated, narrative generally follows linear representations of time. Events happen one after another. It is by assuming an 'end point', from which it surveys all that has gone before, that narrative assumes its figurative dimension and transforms isolated events and successive episodes into a meaningful whole. When patients review their lives for meaningful connections, they frequently discover that 'endings' were actually 'beginnings' and apparent overtures were often 'false starts' or conclusions. This backward reading of events inverts time's 'natural' order, demonstrating how its 'progression' and meaning are far less 'fixed' than we generally assume.

Indeed, our conventional understanding of time is entirely metaphoric. We tend to speak of time as though it were a container for action, an unstoppable river, or distance (Lakoff and Johnson 1980: 41–5). Only when such metaphors fail to mediate what we are actually experiencing, do we cease to take time and its 'passage' for granted. As St Augustine famously remarked, 'What is time? I know full well, until someone asks me.' Existential uncertainty tends to accompany such asking and the patients in this study exhibited a dynamic and mutually influencing triad of temporal sensibility, personal identity and narrative that has attracted comment elsewhere in the context of chronic illness (Charmaz 1991). The metaphors they mobilized are fairly unremarkable. What is noteworthy, however, is the way patients used these metaphors to 'domesticate' unfamiliar or frightening circumstances and events.

During periods of serious illness, time's co-relativity refuses to be ignored. It is well known that the temporal experience of terminally ill people does not coincide with that of the healthy world. For anyone interested in existential or spiritual issues, this co-relativity is particularly interesting for it seems that when conventional understandings of time do 'break down' or fall inadequate before experience, some interest in notions of infinity or eternity may occasionally arise. This is not in the sense of 'conventional' time proceeding without end, but rather as a quality of 'timelessness' or of a potential reality existing 'out of time'. Love or compassion, for example, may be cited as values whose worth exceeds any temporal context, thereby relativising what is happening 'here and now' before a broader and less tangible horizon.

Clearly a detailed philosophy of time lies beyond this book, but there are at least two ways of approaching this observation. Proceeding from the argument that our understanding of time is necessarily approached in finite terms, it can be dismissed as simply fanciful. Death is the condition of our existence and its inevitability is a fundamental defining point for us all. This is the position taken by the philosopher Heidegger (1962) who transforms the question of 'What is time' to 'Who is time' and answers with 'I am my time.' An alternative approach, however, is to ask whether life's ultimate meaning lies not in our own finitude, but in eternity. At this conjunction of temporality, infinity and human nature, however, even philosophical enquiry must end since we do not have the eternal at our disposal from which we may consider time. A theological perspective, however, is not excluded. Theology does not approach the eternal in terms of a methodological requirement, but in terms of faith. Faith, however, is less about the possession of answers—which may anyhow impose an uncomfortable degree of closure or quasi-certainty—than about maintaining an attitude of openness, in this instance, a willingness to consider whether possibilities which are not temporally dependent can be sources of ultimate meaning, or whether patients' experiences of time can be spiritually significant. Although such a proposition is essentially theological, a religious vocabulary is not a necessary prerequisite to its consideration. What matters more is whether the theological exploration is anthropologically grounded. If this is not the case, it will be abstract and meaningless. The following depiction of patients' words and deeds, however, suggests that if anthropology were to exclude a theological perspective from its discussions, an impoverished picture of human experience would result.

Time: familiar friend in unfamiliar circumstances

Time may be something of an enigma or 'familiar stranger' (Fraser 1987), but we all live by temporal metaphors that powerfully and systematically shape our reality. On the whole, patients use conventional metaphors of time (as a resource, distance, motion, appropriateness, container) but, like Victor on 'microwave time', nearly all find themselves struggling with time as something new, threatening and unfamiliar: 'It's all different timing now, in all sorts of ways' (Arthur); 'You're in a different time zone to other people' (Jane).

Hours, days and minutes acquired a new plasticity, becoming unreliable markers and predictors. Eileen, for example, remarked 'I know my time is short, but the days feel so long.' Looking back and fore, time was qualitatively different from its lived experience. Earlier years had flown by, the future approached all too quickly, but the present dragged: 'The days are long but you haven't got as long as you always thought' (Tracey). Often the length of our interview was misjudged. After an hour and a quarter Victor remarked 'Thanks for helping me to pass 20 minutes'. For Debbie, 'It's half-past three? I thought it was about ten to two. I can't tell you how different time feels now, it's weird.' Carla's interview was in early spring but she felt it was 'late in the year for me, a lot of time has already gone.' Mobilizing the metaphor *time as a resource*, Irene's was a fast-diminishing sum whose reserves did not bear contemplation. Victor's time, however, was interest on capital, 'you try and enjoy each day. They say three score years and 10, well I'm seven years on from that, so every day is a bonus.' When time is conceived in terms of spending and saving, losing or giving, the 'worth' of a person becomes entwined with the number of hours others are prepared to devote to their well-being. 'Only one nurse was extra special, she was an absolute gem. She didn't rush in and then, "Bye". We had more of a relationship. The others were all of a rush, rush, rush, rush' (Elsie). Similarly, for Camilla, 'One doesn't tell tales, but there are one or two nurses who just miss the bus. They just aren't with you. Even though they're doing everything right, they're hurrying, thinking about the next job.'

For others, time was the unstoppable Heraclitean river: 'it's passing me by. The future's divorcing me' (Carol). This is *time as motion*, but it does not move at the same pace as for other people: 'you want it frozen, just stopped. You look at your family and they're living a different thing to you. They can't understand the way you look at life now, when you know your time is shot [sic]' (Tracey). Only in fairy tales may an entire court slumber with a sick princess. The schism between Tracey's 'shot' time and that of the healthy world was disorienting for her, 'I'm in limbo ... I might feel better now, but I could go down within a week.' Neither here nor there, limbo suggests the essential ambiguity of transitional time and space, the world of Hermes—ancient guide of souls. Metaphors of time and of liminality, the sense of being on some threshold, are indivisible—much as patients' sensations of time and feelings of control also influence each other. Indeed, all the metaphors that mediate patient experience interpenetrate.

Temporal 'distance'

For many people, the metaphor *time equals distance* helpfully patterned daily life. Their future was uncharted territory but time could be 'stopped' by refusing to 'travel'. As Eunice and Irene respectively explain, 'You're standing still. Treading water. Getting nowhere', 'You don't plan like normal people, just live from day to day.' Any distraction from the furthest outpost—reading, bingo, quizzes, soaps, visits to the day centre—illustrates the use of daily routine to 'bracket out' death (Giddens 1991: 167). The ideal death would be scarcely noticeable—an event, yes, but hopefully not an experience: 'We discussed it fully when I first came out of hospital and when we finished I said, "THAT'S IT", we've discussed it, and now I try not to think about it' (Irene).

Such avoidance is well recognized as a means of coping with imminent mortality (Jarrett *et al.* 1992), illustrating the already commented upon disparity between many patients' notions of a good death (rapid and unexpected) and the tendency of professionals to value a high degree of psychological preparation and inter-familial reconciliation. By mobilizing *time as distance*, however, death is 'upon one' before one has time to realize it. The future has thus been tamed and 'colonization of the future through the assessment and colonization of risk is … a key feature of late-modern self identity' (Seale 1995: 606). This colonization, however, does not equate with the spiritual liberation that stems from recognizing ultimate meaning in the present moment (de Caussade 1981). It may be closer to 'living in the present' as a bizarre form of imprisonment.

Right times and wrong times

Time as a felt degree of appropriateness is not a widely documented metaphor, but a sense of 'right times' and 'wrong times' permeated much patient narrative. The timing of Julia's cardiac arrest, for instance, felt 'all wrong'. Josie was 'broken hearted' when she thought of leaving her children or of her own mother 'losing a second child' (Josie's brother also died in his forties). Nevertheless, Josie maintained 'for me, I feel it's the right time. I'm not afraid. I don't know if something gets released in your brain to help you. I'm not religious, I've no faith, but I just feel I'm going to a peaceful haven.'

Comments from other patients suggest that the means whereby 'right' and 'wrong' times are discerned is not entirely logical. Tracey relied upon her dreams: 'I've been in situations where it's been touch and go. My father's dead, but he told me it wasn't my time to go yet. You do know when your time is up. It's weird, but you do feel it, you just know.' It is not unusual for the psyche to use symbols such as that of the senex, wise old man or father figure, to make available knowledge that is rationally inaccessible (Callanan and Kelley 1992). Debbie also turned for guidance to her late father, 'We're really, really close. He told me before the doctor that it was a tumour. If I've had a hard day, he says "Don't worry, tomorrow will be better".' Eileen was waiting for the 'right time' to die, hoping 'to get some sort of a warning. I hope I'm not just going to pop off like that.' Perhaps her belief that the moment of death would recognizably differ from other times was protective; if presentiments were absent, then so was death. If so, it was a fragile shield easily broached by pain and soon accompanied by what she described as 'troubling thoughts and feelings'. Eileen's desire for a warning is perhaps less unusual than it seems. What she really wanted was for a warning to exist, so that it could be absent—much as a silent siren means danger is not in the air. Irene's logic is, by far, the more typical, 'I want death to be quick, in one's sleep.' Despite the professional 'near-consensus', the official 'script', on the benefits of an aware death (Seale 1995: 609), this study supports a documented preference for 'disregarded dying' or an unanticipated demise during the hours of sleep (Williams 1989).

Throughout our conversation, Eileen's hand rose to a small pendant of a dolphin, a creature whose symbolism has already been commented upon. New that week, Eileen had decided to wear the necklace all the time. In practical terms, this meant until her death. Her practical affairs were resolved, but Eileen wanted time to 'sort things out' with her sister; 'she can't handle it. She doesn't ring me or come to see me. We used to be so close and the more she stays away, the worse it is for me.' At one point, Eileen whispered 'My sister, she collects dolphins. She has lots of little dolphins ... [VERY quietly] ... maybe she can hold one at my funeral.' Although the symbol transcends differences of time and location, Eileen's need to connect with her sister was immediate. She wore the pendant constantly and so 'ever now'. Perhaps courage, as much as time, was needed. Appropriately supported, perhaps Eileen could have risked rejection. One suspects that without some overture to her sister, last chances were being missed and no time would ever feel 'right' for her to die. It is difficult to witness patients exposing themselves to emotional danger. As well as not wanting to see a patient hurt further, Eileen's situation can bring to mind carers' own 'unfinished business'. Dissuasion from taking risks, however, disrespects the gravity of the patient's situation. Heart piercing pain may merely be exchanged for a smothering depression which may, in the final analysis, prove more debilitating. Paradoxically, may not even unpalatable truths have something of healing in them, simply because they are a place from which to begin again, where beginnings imply not distance/time, but the more real/depth? 'The Latin verb *ferre* means to bear, to carry and suffer derives from it, with the prefix 'sub' meaning 'under'. ... In contrast to the word 'suffer', such terms as 'affliction', 'grief', and 'depression' all bring images of weight bearing down. Grief is derived from *gravare*. Only when we suffer in the full sense of the word do we *carry* the weight. ... The only valid cure for any kind of depression lies in the acceptance of real suffering and real suffering will lead us to seek the appropriate help. Thus we begin to build the "undercarriage" of suffering upon which the superstructure of our lives may securely rest' (Luke 1987: 103). Furthermore, Luke continues, 'however great our efforts may be to achieve this conscious attitude to suffering, we cannot succeed without an awareness that, in spite of apparent senselessness, there is always an implicit universal meaning even in the carrying of small miseries ... one is released into a sense of meaning ... it is as though we become aware of a new dimension. Meaning has entered the experience' (Luke 1987: 107).

As conventional temporality becomes increasingly extenuated, psychological explanations tend to overlook certain aspects of experience. Luke's 'new dimension' certainly lures her beyond her impeccable Jungian training. Although his final statement is curiously reminiscent of philosophical notions of being and non-being, Fred describes events more exhaustively considered by theology than by any other discipline: 'There is a higher life form, you can call him God, call him Buddha, whatever. I do pray. I take great comfort from that. If someone interrupts me I just say, "Excuse me I'm having a meditation" and shut my eyes and go back. I'm in my body but I'm not in my body.' Although most patients used temporal metaphors to bolster feelings of control, to reassert the 'being' of time, Fred meditated to loosen its conventional strictures. Similarly, Carla escaped from anxiety and her habitual chain smoking through painting. So occupied, she 'lost track of time' and pondered issues of ultimate meaning in ways that expose the superficiality of much of the 'companionship' she otherwise experienced: 'Some people talk such a lot of rubbish. There are only so many answers to "what a pretty night-dress". I don't want to talk about the weather. I want to talk about my painting. I need to talk about it. When I'm painting I'm away from everything in the colour. People are deeper than you think. I don't want to talk about trivial things any more. I want to talk about things that interest me; spiritualism, about how my death might be, about how long I might have left. I'm not saying I want to be deep all the time, I can talk at the other level too, but it isn't what interests me now.'

Both the painting and the meditation destabilize conventional perceptions of time to bring comforting patterns of meaning to the trials of illness. Both are concerned with encounter, for Carla and Fred speak as recipients. Similarly, Eileen described her attempts to find some peace: 'When I got ill I started to pray and go back to church. It has helped; sometimes it's more two way.' Such comforting and tentative 'disclosures' of meaning, whether via art, meditation, conversation or religious participation can confer events with a significance or 'rightness' that defies logic or 'common sense'. When listening to patients give account of baffling phenomena, carers are well advised to remember Yeats' (1982: 81) injunction: 'I being poor, have only my dreams; I have spread them under your feet, Tread softly because you tread on my dreams.'

Proximity to death not only undermines taken-for-granted sensations of time, the conventional strictures relating to presence also invite contemplation. It is to this end, not to make any point about the supernatural, that Gregory's experience is recounted. As his health declined, one memory repeatedly surfaced. Feeling rationally confounded, Gregory symbolically defers to feminine wisdom, to Sophia, by citing his mother: 'I had a friend who was convinced beyond all doubt that there was a second life. I found myself saying, "I envy you your faith". I did, because he was so convinced. Well, at about this time, I had this, I can't tell you, it was a dream probably, but I had this vision of him walking up an avenue of trees towards me saying, "I told you, Gregory". I just pictured it all very strongly in my mind. I don't know what it was, but it was very strong. It coincided with him suddenly dying while he was away on holiday, aged 47. That was 25 years ago. My mother said I had a vision, but I don't know.'

Gregory was also mystified by questions of 'Why now?'—Why emerge unscathed from active service and enjoy perfect health until retirement, only to nurse his wife until she no longer recognized him? Why, when he finally had some leisure, should he lose his sight and become terminally ill? Any attempt to find meaning in the human condition is indissoluble from a theological consideration of time, for 'Why me?' is entwined almost to a point of tautology with 'Why now?' Debbie, for example, found that 'Lots of people say "Oh, why you Debbie? You've just got married. You've just qualified. This is your time, Debbie."'

Just as wisdom is not simply a matter of accumulated experience, the relationship between time, circumstance and identity defies external logical criteria. The natural tendency to find the death of a young adult or child more tragic than that of an old person, for instance, curiously evaluates a life's worth by its unspent potential, its non-being. Carers sometimes feel greater sympathy for young patients, forgetting that for someone like Elsie, the right time to die is not chronologically determined: 'Talking to you now, I don't think I'm 83. I could be 53, for all that matters. I don't feel any different. It makes me sad because I would like to go on to over a hundred.' As Gregory wryly observed, 'it's a natural phenomena that we've all got used to, waking up in the morning.'

Regrets and mistakes: 're-membering' the past

'What a long distance lies between an act and its consequences' (Murdoch 1979: 345). Sifting through past events can expose the inappropriateness of actions once considered 'right'. Claude and his wife were childless—a decision that now drew tears. Fear and regret framed the future Elspeth envisaged for her daughter: 'She's never been on one date in her whole life. Friends who went to college made lots of new friends, but Gina didn't go. I wish we'd made her; it might have helped her blossom. Her friends get fewer and fewer as they marry.' Although younger people are vulnerable to anguished realizations, from the vantage point of old age, past actions and missed opportunities may invoke a sadness, even shame, whose reasons are imperceptible to younger carers or simply lie beyond their ken. Some of the older men, for example, may have more comfortably shared war-time memories in the presence of a male (or more experienced) interviewer. Gregory was not alone in hinting at troubling sexual recollections: 'I was a bit wild. You can imagine a navy ship— all those men coming into town, with the women. I was in the marines and they don't teach you to be a namby-pamby. Hundreds and thousands were taught the same. But when you are young, you do stupid things. It took me a year to settle down.' Given the predominance of female over male carers and a taboo many older men may feel in sharing "men's talk" with women, the case for increasing a masculine presence in hospice perhaps merits attention.

Particular incidents or 'skellingtons', as Arthur called them, may not be so much the focus of regret, as a nagging feeling of not having lived one's 'real life'. Tolstoy (1996: 152) famously captures the sentiment when the dying Ivan Illych asks 'What if my whole life has really been wrong?' Similar feelings receive a theological echo, an openness to possibility, from Hazel, 'I shan't live so very much longer and all these happenings, they make you review your life. I needed more spiritual experience than I ever had. I missed the mark and scattered my energies. Now they are all dying out and I must find something to fill the gap. That's a crude way, I suppose, of saying I'm still on the spiritual path, or try to be.'

Under the maxim 'forgiveness frees us', Longaker (1997: 93) suggests a number of exercises for 'making connections, healing relationships and letting go'. Such opportunities, she argues, persist even in times of crises. Carla illustrates the argument thus: 'Sometimes I just sit and think of all the people who will die today, without any idea of what's coming. At least I have some time to think.' Peace of mind, however, does not always depend on personal effort. Some never experience a resolution of their troubles, even after years of struggle. For others, such as Josie, peace comes as an unexpected but welcome benediction, 'I just can't say why I'm not frightened. After my second radio-therapy treatment I was waiting for the porter and I was so calm. When I lay abed, I just thought through everything and I was calm, relaxed, I can't explain it.'

Theologians are not people with privileged access to extraordinary experiences. A theological statement simply tries to explain an experience such as Josie's at its most fundamental level and can only be judged by its apparent success. Tillich, for example, maintains that 'every moment of time reaches into the eternal … the eternal "now" provides for us a temporal "now" … Not everybody and nobody all the time is aware of this "eternal" now in the temporal "now". But sometimes it breaks powerfully into our consciousness and gives us the certainty of the eternal … [of entering into] the divine rest' (Tillich 1963: 111). It is interesting to contemplate Carol's experience in the same light. Despite her total paralysis, she experienced 'a strange but understandable change of heart about nearly everything that bothered me in life. I feel a greater power than me is at work, I feel free. All that has come about because of St Christopher's. Before admission, I was twisted and knotted about my dependence, my sister's health and her efforts to give me as normal a life as possible. There's such a special spirit here. I can only liken it to being struck by something beautiful I didn't expect or think existed—the safety, the knowledge, the loving care.' Good palliative care, as Carol's appreciation shows, is good spiritual care. In Hasidic style, the theologian Buber (1947: 14) makes a similar point: 'A man inspired by God once went out from the creaturely realms into the vast waste. There he wandered till he came to the gates of the mystery. He knocked. From within came the cry: "What do you want here?" He said, "I have proclaimed your praise in the ears of mortals but they were deaf to me. So I came to you that you yourself may hear me and reply." "Turn back" came the cry from within. "Here is no ear for you. I have sunk my hearing in the deafness of mortals." ... [True address from God] directs man into the place of lived speech, where the voices of the creatures grope past one another, and in their very missing of one another, succeed in reaching the eternal partner.'

Plural temporality

There is a sense in which our understanding of time depends upon our descriptions of the things about which we care. The making present of these things and our interpretation of them are indivisible. Time, therefore, is not simply available in quantitative or linear terms with minutes, hours and days fitting neatly within each other. Time has a tensive, qualitative dimension and multiple temporalities co-exist. If, for example, tomorrow is my birthday, time drags. Unfortunately, if I must also have a tooth extraction, time flies by. It is hardly surprising if illness distorts temporal perceptions and Tracey expresses its ambiguities thus: 'I look forward to Christmas with the family, then I don't want it to come. I think, "Am I going to be here Christmas coming?"'

Taking death as time's defining point does not exclude notions of multiple temporality. To explore the human quest for meaning and its spiritual implications, however, one must consider whether human time is lived against the allure of eternity, in this instance, whether patients ever locate themselves against, or search for a temporal frame infinitely wider than that of their own life. Furthermore, if seen in such a perspective, do patients' experiences acquire a greater depth of meaning, are they seen in a more comforting light? A famous sparrow flight through an open window into a brightly lit hall and out again on the other side illustrates the common presentiment of there existing a time that is not one's own, a time that extends beyond the limits of one's past and future. From the perspective of the self, human time is the bright and familiar hall, the darkness is wholly 'other'. Should there be nothing 'other' than that which is finite, however, Elspeth's concern to locate her life in a wider perspective, her belief in a wider dispersion of presence and her desire for continuation will inevitably come to a point where they are irrelevant: 'I think nothing can be completely destroyed. If you smash a brick it becomes dust and goes into the earth and it's the same for bodies. I used to think that if you'd been an influence on people you carried on. The genes do go on, except I don't have grandchildren and some families die out altogether.'

'O Lord, let something remain' is an ancient lament. The reach of human life, however, resists our notions of existential justice. Gregory struggled to understand why his maternal grandparents died in their forties when his paternal grandparents, after burying their thirteen children, lived until their nineties: 'How the hell can there be so much difference between the two? Oh God, It's incredible. You look into the fairness of it, but run into a maze. It's impossible to understand.' Not all problems are susceptible to logic and the whole person is not characterized simply by rationality. Gregory's 'maze' is similar to Carla's mandala. Contemplation of neither yields any 'answer' to life's confounding circumstances, but each springs from and fosters deepening levels of awareness. Any profound realization, be it of mortality or fecundity, is a process of coming to 'be', as well as of coming to 'know'. Gregory simply reveals the imprint of mystery on the human condition and the longing of finite creatures for ultimate security. Before his illness he thought 'dying was like having two buttons: one for death and one for life. When it's ended, just press the death button. I've realized that it's not like that. It goes on longer. If I said I wasn't afraid, it wouldn't be true. I don't know what to expect. I've no indication of the future. I'd like to believe in it, but I don't know. We'll just have to wait and see.' Although reflecting on her experiences of pregnancy, Mary expresses similar processes of becoming and a similar sense of liminality: 'I never could believe that I could produce a child. The whole idea of having this thing that grows inside of you, that you've made ... it just felt wonderful. I felt on a great threshold there.'

The individual who contemplates the co-relativity of human life and eternity is open to notions of a transcendent order. Even if, as in Edwin's case, his response is one of refutation, such contemplations inevitably expose him to the possibility of some ultimate purpose and meaning in life: 'It might sound stupid, but I believed for a long time that Jesus was a spaceman sent to help us. But there can't be somebody up there, because if you look into the sky it goes on for infinity. Besides, how can someone so good allow children to die, money worries, war?' As Edwin struggled with notions of ultimate love and justice, the religious metaphors he retained from childhood (heaven as a place; the existence of a fair 'moral economy') buckled under the weight of his suffering. His substitution of 'Jesus as spaceman', however, is both original and beautiful. 'Saying' more than he 'knew', he was surely unaware of any symmetry between his novel metaphor and Teilhard de Chardin's declaration that 'In Jesus, the universe before us assumes a face and heart' (Heaney 1984: 88). Although Judith also pondered on infinity, her thoughts did not result in nihilism, but in a consolation that echoes earlier more classical abandonments that may be summarized: 'What does it matter whether I live or I die for I belong to God?'. She said, 'I am going to die, no matter what. If you believe in eternity—always has been and always will be—a year or two doesn't make much difference. What I mean is, if you die at twenty or fifty or even one hundred, if you're looking at time as never ending, it's nothing you know.'

It is experience that grounds rhetoric, not vice versa: 'You know the words "God is Love"? Well, where is he in all this? It's nonsense' (Elsie). It was not unusual for patients to react angrily when their conceptions of how God 'should' behave (again, often based on metaphors they carried from childhood) were shattered. Paradoxically, however, Jane's fury at the apparent absence of a fair 'moral economy' demonstrates her commitment to the ultimate value of justice. The metaphor may have collapsed, but her anger expresses the continuing influence and desire for the good that it disclosed: 'Why me? It doesn't make sense. This is a living nightmare. It should be somebody evil, but it doesn't happen to them. I've never been religious but I've sort of believed there's something better. But I can't see a reason for me getting this. If there is a God up there, he's wicked.' Elspeth demonstrates a similar commitment to ultimate values combined with a strong desire to retain her personal integrity: 'I don't believe in murder or hitting people but I'm not religious and I don't think you should start asking for help at the last minute.'

Questions of meaning—'Why me?' or 'Why now?'—are indivisible from temporal metaphor. Our understanding of ourselves shapes our understanding of time and our understanding of time moulds our sense of self. Patients' struggles with such questions and with their altered perceptions of time point to an inevitable tension in the human condition for 'There is no other way of judging time than to see it in the light of the eternal. In order to judge something, one must be partly within it, partly out of it. If we were totally within time, we would not be able to elevate ourselves in prayer, meditation and thought, to the eternal. We would be creatures of time like all other creatures and could not ask the question of the meaning of time. But, as men, we are aware of the eternal to which we belong and from which we are estranged by the burden of time' (Tillich 1963: 103). It is in living and contemplating this tension that anthropological vision is extended to a spiritual horizon. For Hindus, 'wrong action' is not that of living in time, but in believing that nothing exists outside time. In forgetting eternity, one is consumed by time, mistaking it for the ultimate reality. Illusion stems not from living in history, but in regarding it as the sum total of reality.

In moves entirely commensurate with contemporary and post-modern destabilizations of certainty, serious illness means that time may no longer be

relied upon. Insecurity and doubt, however, may not be signs of spiritual iner-
tia, but of an awakening to the disconcerting tensions between human time
and infinity. In a context where relationships are strained and people are
struggling to find meaning, the vulnerability of the conventional stories in
which our lives are couched is exposed. Existential insecurity is invoked and
far-reaching questions are raised. Nevertheless, without wishing to undermine
their suffering and difficulties, there are patients for whom experiences of
temporal estrangement seem to result in novel convictions and penetrative
insights that may be regarded as spiritually significant. Some patients seem to
realize in a new way the 'kind of story' they would, or do, inhabit.

The infinite perspective: core values and the seer

All spiritual traditions claim that the fundamental values for living emanate from
an ultimate or eternal dimension. It is the responsibility of the seer to draw attention to this dimension. In archaic society he was defined by his ability to detach
himself from profane time, magically re-entering original or 'Great Time' by imi-
tating exemplary acts or by reciting certain adventures (Eliade 1957: 23). He
would then 'return' to his own people with increased wisdom and an augmented
vision. It was his responsibility to benefit the wider community by providing
explanations, warnings and encouragement. The authority of his pronounce-
ments rested in his cosmogenic perspective—a direct result of his willingness to
abandon his conventional self and conventional temporality. Generally speaking,
however, modern man resists the developmental processes of the seer. Notions of
'self but non-self' are confounding and various activities promote illusions of
mastery over any personal surrender: time is 'killed', 'escaped from' or becomes a
period of heightened intensity to be summoned at will.

The main point here, however, is that impending mortality sometimes causes people to reappraise their priorities and concerns to such a degree, and with
such a strong desire for others to see likewise, that it is not an exaggeration to
compare them with the seers of old. Throughout the interviews many patients
appealed, sometimes incongruously, to what might be termed core values:
'Never ignore another human being's cry for help' (Fred); 'Treat people as you
like to be treated yourself. If you talk about people don't talk bad' (Eunice);
'Do as you would be done by. Be kind, be nice, be patient to people' (Camilla).
Debbie and Tracey also wanted people to value themselves without guilt: 'Now
I see life at a deeper level, my whole attitude is different. It's the first time I've
ever put myself first. It's not about being selfish, it's about being at peace'
(Debbie); 'Take time out to build yourself up. Let someone else do something
nice for you. Treat yourself good. If you don't, you only get to pay back at the
end' (Tracey).

Gregory best illustrates the quasi-prophetic urgency of such pronounce-ments. He seemed to despair at what he called the 'blindness' of others (although he was literally blind) and their inability to 'see' what really matters in life. Expressing what many would regard as a universal spiritual truth, Gregory argues that love is the highest activity to have arisen from creation: 'I hear silly little arguments and think: My God, what a waste of time. If only they knew. Why don't they realize? [louder and with feeling] People are wast-ing precious moments, wasting their precious hours arguing and having rows. How silly, how stupid. Why can't they see? [nearly shouting, gesticulating] It is so trivial. The most important thing is to try and be kind, try and be thought-ful. [slowly and deliberately articulated] In my opinion, love is the essence of everything.'

Gregory was not alone in linking his appreciation of *time as a precious resource* with qualities of human interaction. Jane found she had become 'more tolerant of people' and answered her own question, 'Why have argu-ments? There's not enough time for it.' Carol also expressed novel liberating priorities. Her talk of losing and finding mobilizes a metaphor articulated in all spiritual traditions. She uses it to disclose the paradox of finding freedom and personal growth in spite of advancing paralysis. Like Gregory, she too expresses the core value of love: 'I used to feel guilty for being divorced twice and a failure, but these feelings are going rapidly. Being ill has fit things into perspective for me. You can see the sense of freedom in my poems. I've had to lose myself to find myself. I feel well being in throwing off the shackles of materialism. I've learned to love people for what they are and not to compart-mentalize; not to put anyone's worth in terms of their status.'

Carol's failed relationships no longer exist simply in relation to one another. Her experience of illness has brought her a new vision, a new horizon against which to measure herself. In their new and expansive context, her life's painful 'truths', her divorces and sense of failure, surrender something of their bite. Interpreted theologically, 'what has happened has happened and remains so for all eternity', but 'the meaning of the facts can be changed by the eternal, and the name of this change is the experience of "forgiveness"' (Tillich 1963: 109). Inevitably, paradox (finding in losing), metaphor and imagery (throwing away her shackles) are the 'tools' of a language of spirit. Only by using images taken from time may we express our understanding of the eternal and dis-cover its implications for the here and now.

The deeper meaning of events is rarely revealed by a superficial exploration. Carol's situation, for example, could be approached simply in terms of a per-sonal tragedy. Every gesture, act of speech or personal exchange, however, is part of a complex symbol system and contains many depths of meaning.

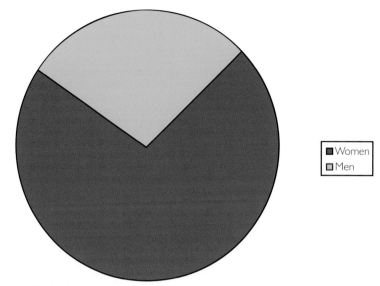

Plate 1 Distributions of participants by gender. (See Fig. 3.1.)

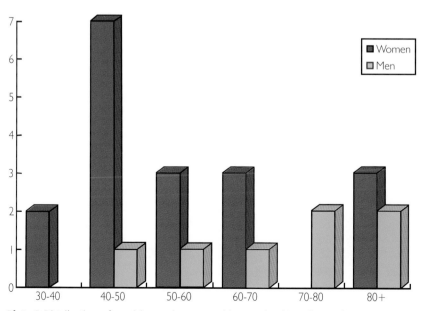

Plate 2 Distribution of participants by age and by gender. (See Fig. 3.2.)

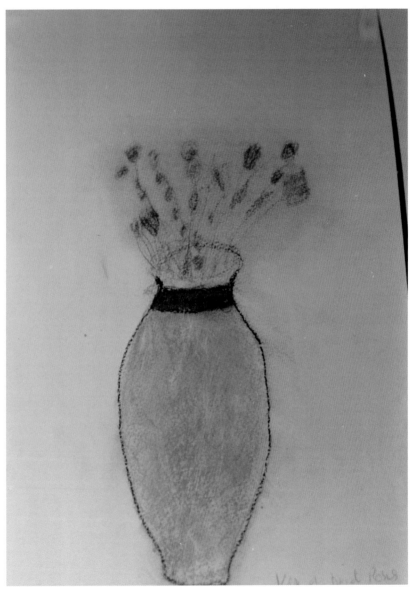

Plate 3 Vase of dried flowers. (See Fig. 7.1.)

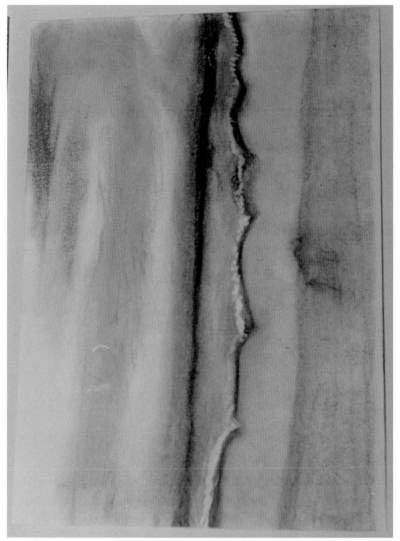

Plate 4 On the beach. (See Fig. 7.2.)

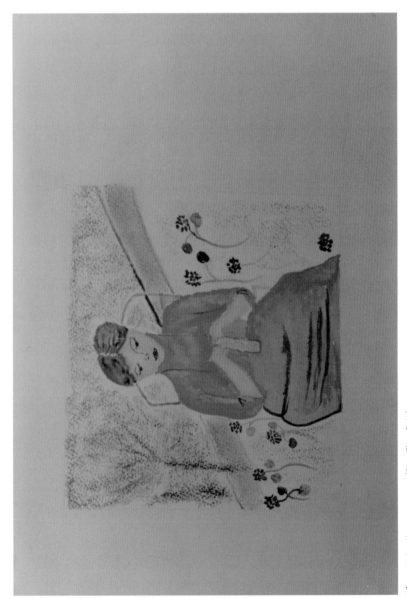

Plate 5 Sewing woman. (See Fig. 9.1.)

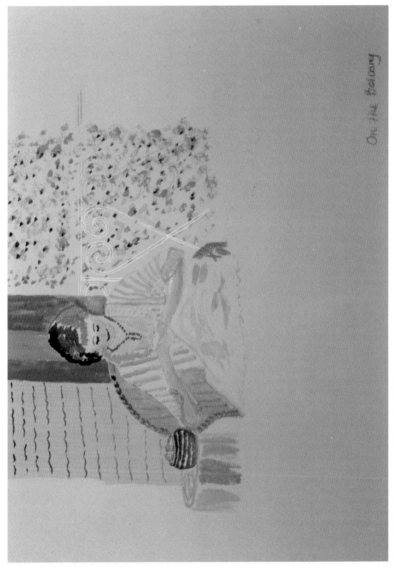

Plate 6 On the balcony. (See Fig. 9.2.)

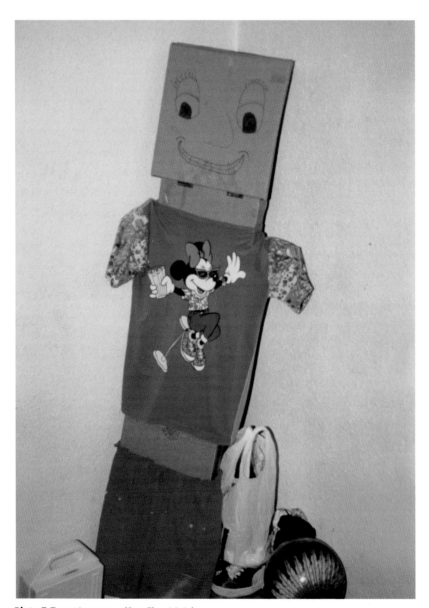

Plate 7 Tracey's statue. (See Fig. 11.1.)

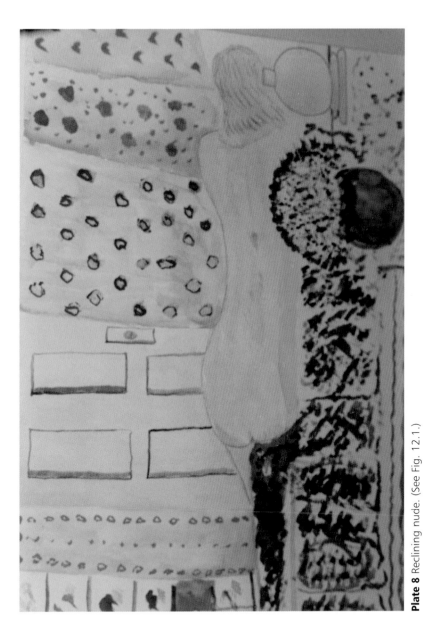

Plate 8 Reclining nude. (See Fig. 12.1.)

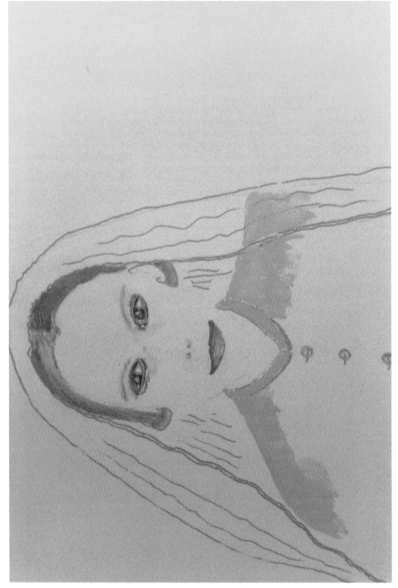

Plate 9 Carla's bride. (See Fig. 12.2.)

Carol, Gregory, Jane and others show us that patients do not have to use theological or religious language to express recognizably spiritual concerns. Consequently, we are primarily interested in the spiritual significance mediated by each symbol, not its specific form. Eunice explains the point: 'You may call it one thing and me another. Some call it this, some call it that, some worship this, some worship that, but when you boil it down, it's the one God.' This does not mean that all statements are of equal value, but points to a discerning critical realism. It would be presumptuous to claim to know what Eunice means when she says 'God', but there is a sense in which the term is a religious cipher for what is ultimately unknowable to finite creatures. Certainly, as Eunice realized, the final word on matters of infinity is not ours to give because 'the more you dive in, the deeper it goes and the further you can divulge'.

Final comments

Listening to patients talk about time is like hearing them describe Fraser's (1987) 'familiar stranger'. Their conventional understanding is challenged in ways that reveal much about what it is like to face death, to feel socially dislocated or to struggle with 'wrong times'. Perhaps unsurprisingly, many people try to re-establish feelings of control through temporal metaphor that keeps the future at bay. Perceptions of time are nevertheless inextricably linked with the human quest for meaning and identity. For certain patients, 'Why me?' was virtually interchangeable with 'Why now?' so that their personal explorations, either implicitly or explicitly ask, 'Am I related to anything infinite?' This is simply another way of asking 'What is the meaning of (my) life?' Closed philosophical systems take death as their defining point but given all that patients say and experience it seems unreasonable to deny every intimation of an infinite perspective or ultimate horizon. This is a question of spiritual awareness that, at the very least, should remain open.

Many people, maybe most, die without exhibiting any sign of caring about ultimate values. Nevertheless, human temporality and spirituality are inextricably interwoven with altered perceptions of time sometimes accompanied by an awakening spiritual awareness. Distinctions of healing and curing are not new and the spiritual traditions each support the possibility of positive transformation up to, often beyond, life's final moments. 'Dying is never a hopeless state' (Longaker 1997: 157) because 'forgiveness', as defined by Tillich, is a 'knowledge' that evades temporal strictures. Carers may not conjure up such insights. It is, however, reasonable to want to help patients to 'clear a space', from which time's fracturing experiences are glimpsed against a wider and infinitely loving horizon.

Chapter 7

Marginality and liminality: metaphors of the edge or the way?

Mud may be dirt when it gets on the carpet (Douglas 1978: 2), but clear lines of demarcation do not always exist between one state and another. Metaphors of marginality and liminality provide alternative 'orderings' or meanings to events that initially may appear synonymous. Both are characterized by loss or separation, by uncertainty and grief, by memories of one's former self. In experiences of marginality, individuals tend to feel pushed towards some fringe. Elsie, for example identified with 'those people you see on the streets, drinkers. I used to hate seeing them in parks and gardens. But, thinking about it, they're so dejected aren't they? We judge them too much when we don't know what's happened. I mean, I'm like that now, on the edge, with the dregs.'

Similar feelings often accompany liminal experiences, but liminality is primarily about a deep inner process of becoming, rather than experiences of exclusion. Coming from limen, the Latin for doorway or threshold, liminality implies a borderline state. One is betwixt and between, if only for a moment, as when is leaving or entering a room. Liminal and marginal states are not necessarily opposed; 'frontier' is a good unitive term. Nevertheless, despite Elsie's plea for understanding, 'to define oneself as marginal is to define oneself in relation to someone else's centre; it is to accept another's version of how things are. In that sense it may be quite disempowering and in itself alienating. To have one's base and focus on the margins is to have a view of the present and the past, but what of the future? Threshold implies future. To be between here and there is to live in the faith that there is a future. To choose between here and there is to live in the faith it will be a better future' (Ward and Wild 1996: 30). Liminality may feel chaotic and dangerous but it also symbolizes creativity and power. A new authoritative meaning always emerges from its disorder. The emotional costs of submitting to this state, however, are high and involve 'letting go' of what was once taken for granted. Nevertheless, if there is any sense of direction it is predominantly forward and not 'out'. Despite her near total paralysis, Carol's sense of 'stepping out of an unhappy place into a freedom to develop my own feelings and attitudes' can thus be approached in terms of liminality.

Invocation of the limen may imply a 'beyond', but it is generally vague and ill defined. Those in a liminal state are rarely as confident as Carol. They tend towards to sudden shifts in confidence and heightened emotions so that 'simple' events can appear deeply significant, never to be forgotten. Hermes, transporter of souls, is a classically liminal figure and night time is his element. When one is neither fully awake nor completely asleep, one is in a liminal state. Mutualities of time and identity can become strained and troubling insecurities emerge. Consequently, Irene would always take a sleeping tablet; 'If I can go off to sleep in that first half hour, I don't have time to think about it and mull things over.' Critical questions of meaning—'Who am I?', 'Where am I going to?', 'Why is this happening to me?', 'Why now?'—acquire greater urgency during the night, naturally leading to areas of thought and feeling that are more easily submerged by daytime activities. Angela, the groomed poised and helpful vicar's wife by day, weeping and frightened by night, has already been commented upon.

Although liminal and marginal experiences are regular bedfellows, one is no guarantor of the other. Meaning differs radically according to which of the two metaphors dominates the patterning of experience. Ward and Wild (1996) make a useful analogy with natural deserts or the wilderness. For the exile, life in the desert is reluctantly taken up and generally perceived as a marginal existence. Nevertheless, deserts can be places of refuge. Hostile environments are certainly essential to the survival of the planet and every life passes through difficult but necessary transitions. We naturally draw back from the unfamiliar, from the strange and dangerous 'deserts' between 'here' and 'there', even when they contain a liminal potential. In ways absent to a purely marginal experience, transition can be a threshold to new perceptions. Again, the seer is a relevant figure. Only after experiencing the wilderness does his vision differ from those who remained at home. Only after Sadie experienced disability personally could she see that 'all those years when I thought I wasn't being condescending to people in wheelchairs, I was. It's only just hit me now.'

Apparently, as many as one in three people today consider themselves to have experienced moments of expanded spiritual awareness (Hay 1990). This awareness seems to resemble some of the conditions of liminality. Generally unexpected, it may even challenge conventional sensory perception. Although individuals may feel powerless to control any events surrounding or leading up to their expanded awareness they are usually left with a new sense of purpose or direction. Hazel's described childhood experience is an extreme instance: 'I had a curious smell about my body like a pine forest. I kept taking baths but it lasted for 10 days. Everything looked wonderful. For 10 days I saw everything in a golden light and everything seemed to go excellently. It was so clear that it wasn't coming from me, it was coming to me. But the awful thing was that it faded. In a sort of a way, I was taken up by the experience. It was an idea expressed in the iridescent. It was new to me, but not really new.'

There is a sense of encounter here, of being 'taken up' by a knowledge that is non-conceptual—hence the resort to imagery. The authenticity of accounts such as this, or of patients such as Fred who meditated, Eileen, Mary, Carol or Judith who were comforted by prayer and Irene who was calmed by contemplating her place in a cosmos where 'nothing can be totally destroyed' plus the many hundreds of others collected by Hay, may be judged only by their consequences. Hazel felt her encounter acted as 'an opening, because I then transferred my thinking towards the spiritual life rather than the intellectual.' If she, armed with a theological vocabulary, found articulating her experience and its meaning difficult, how much stronger is the case for paying attention to the images and metaphors of all patients.

Although many patients tended to describe their situation in either predominantly marginal or liminal patterns, these could fluctuate at different times in the same person and circumstance was no predictor of meaning. Of two people with apparently similar difficulties, one could express feelings of liminality, the other of marginality. As two of Carla's paintings (Figs 7.1 and 7.2) illustrate, the language of liminality, of threshold and possibility, as well as of pain and confusion, does not necessarily require a religious vocabulary. (Perhaps it is worth noting as an aside, that while I recorded Carla's comments about her paintings, in no sense did I attempt to interpret or 'analyse' her work for her.)

'Vase of Dried Flowers' (Fig. 7.1) was produced at about the time when Carla described herself as peripheral to her family and friends, existing at the perimeter of many circles. The blue-grey, she explained, spoke of her depression and sadness, the red and black, of her pain and anger. Certainly, the image is striking: the confinement affected by the black border, the compression and violence suggested by the tight red collar, the mal-proportion of stunted flowers to vase. Interestingly, the flowers are dried and thus an inauthentic life form, whilst their colour and haze suggest a miasmic rawness. Standing alone and so without grounding, relativising perspective or any sense of alternative, this is a bold, despairing and anguished statement. Conventionally symbolized by the bowl or vase, the anima is here tragically displayed by a woman who found herself at the margins of her family and her physical capabilities. Small wonder that when speaking of the red collar, Carla mimed herself as being strangled.

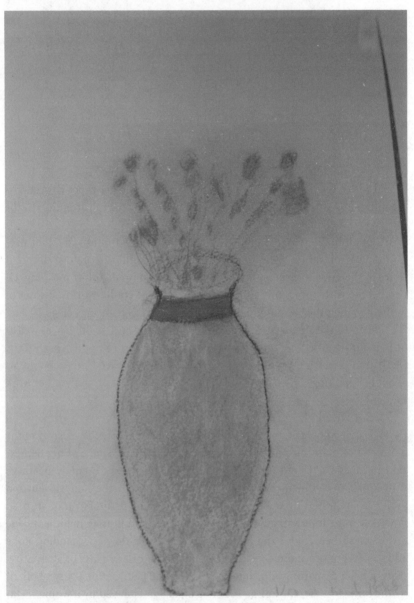

Figure 7.1 Vase of dried flowers. (See Colour Plate 3.)

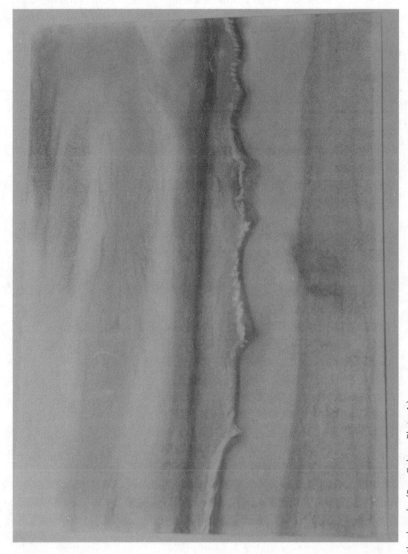

Figure 7.2 On the beach. (See Colour Plate 4.)

Although painful, disturbing and ultimately more fundamental in its challenge, Carla's painting of an isolated beach (Fig. 7.2) is a more enigmatic image. Spilling over the edges of the paper, the vista suggests immediate, dark and terrifying possibilities. The brightest horizon seems too distant and impersonal to offer comfort to anyone standing on the beach. Nevertheless, a sense of expansion, of frightening potential, rather than of compression, characterizes this work whose clear sequential motif of sand, sea and sky infuses a dynamic quality, as opposed to the stasis of the dried flowers. The furthest horizon both draws and tantalizes the viewer for it is unclear whether this is sunrise or sunset. The emboldened shore and skyline possess an absolute and final quality and the faint little dog, miniaturized by the ocean he faces, speaks of the instinctive quaking of the finite, the physical, before such enormity. He too is quite alone, without a substitute. Unlike the vase, however, he exists in a recognizable and epic landscape.

This painting is the more authoritative of the two works for viewers are enjoined are to consider their own vantage point. Whereas the vase calls forth a subject-to-object mode of relating, the rapport encouraged by Fig. 7.2 is from subject to subject, for the scene is witnessed from within the picture, from higher up the beach. To really see such a picture invites a painful contemplation of inevitability, of boundary and transition. The viewer cannot fail to realize that one day they too must stand powerless at the water's edge. In short, this painting both expresses and invokes an awareness of liminality.

In summary, metaphors of liminality and marginality challenge personal identity. Either may be experienced as painful, but the liminal situation harbours a dynamic and potential that eludes the purely marginal. Although experiences of liminality lie beyond an individual's control, they sometimes induce an expanded consciousness of what life is ultimately about and what really matters. The potential and range of either metaphor to mediate ultimate or spiritual concerns will become more apparent as the prism (Fig. 6.1) is further constructed. Their appreciation is particularly relevant to its eighth facet concerning the mediating influence of metaphors of estrangement for terminally ill people.

Chapter 8

Metaphors of control

Introduction

Personal control over one's life is significantly correlated with self-esteem and levels of anxiety. Autonomy and the ability to manipulate or influence circumstance are consistent and significant predictors of quality of life (Lewis 1982). Many patients, however, spoke in terms suggesting helplessness and impotency; of being carried along on what Debbie called 'a roller coaster ride'; Mary sighed 'I used to be "Mum" but now I'm just a rag doll to be washed and dressed'; Tracey likened her cancer to 'an alien taking me over'. Although Sadie feared she would 'explode like a bomb', even this unpredictable force was no guarantee against feeling 'like a puppet on a string'. Claude evokes the grip of an unfeeling but efficient machine: 'My GP reacted very quickly. Everything worked like clockwork: GP to specialist, specialist to hospital, and therapy to clinic … [voice breaking and fading to a whisper]. Remarkably efficient the way it ran.'

Helplessness before destiny—'if it's got your number on it' (Elsie) and life as an implacable lottery—a matter of 'taking your chances' (Irene) or of 'waiting for the penny to fall' (Arthur) were common themes. Patients mourned their vanishing options and impossible 'choices' were rejected: 'My condition is fatal. I haven't got a second chance, so I'm afraid I've got no choices, and that's final' (Gregory); 'The doctor can't do much but slow it down, so I've got no choices, have I?' (Edwin).

To be powerful is to be recognized, to feel as though one matters to other people; one counts for something in their eyes (May 1972: 99). Tracey's 'choice' fulfils these requirements but, unusually, it signifies compulsion and exhaustion, not potency: 'Sometimes I think, leave me … I just want to lay down and be ill. Just leave me. Give me a rest. I don't wanna smile. I don't wanna get up and make the effort. I just wanna lay down. But, as I said, my life has to be my kids, so that has to be my choice.' Sadie illustrates a more typical drift away from feelings of significance and control: 'Who needs me now, really? Doing what? Before, I ran this ladies darts league. I ran the lot and I liked that control. I had to be strong to hear myself speaking. But now, I can't do a thing the way I used to.'

There is little of the nutritive or integrative features of power (May 1972) here, but an understandable tendency to focus upon redundant competitive forms of behaviour. Distressing losses of control were often spoken of in manipulative terms. Control could no longer be exerted 'over' the emotions, the environment, the body or relationships. Claude, for example, wept even as he described breaking down with two of his friends: 'It's too bad that I don't have control. My father was in this state when he was dying. He lost control whenever you talked to him, just started crying.' Elsie bemoaned her recent inability to check her temper: 'Before, I hardly ever said a swear word. Now, you should be behind me, I'm blasting away like mad. You're so angry, you damn and blast.' As a regional manager, Fred used his declining professional capacity to monitor the progress of his illness more than his physical symptoms: 'Sometimes, I'd have a good day at work. Sometimes, I'd have a bad day. In the end, I lost control of all my territory and I could never work on my own. They wouldn't let me. I applied for early retirement because I was bored. It was granted in three weeks. Unfortunately, I really went downhill after that.'

For many patients, the prospect of becoming a drain on the emotional and financial resources of family and friends could evoke powerful feelings of guilt: 'I don't want to go on living if I get very incapacitated. I'm a nuisance' (Hazel). Bernard's stoic veneer only thinly disguised his sense of being a 'burden' rather than a purposive agent: 'I was very unsure about where I was going to be put. I think they have arranged I'm going to live in an old people's home ... but ... well, perhaps it's best all round, for everybody, if I called it a day now.' Making the same point, but from a different angle, Irene and Judith—mothers of older children, were relieved to be 'no longer really needed' by their families (Irene). They were pleased not to be leaving an 'unfair' workload for their partners. Carol's feelings about her illness were those of 'devastation and disbelief' but she found comfort in believing 'if it had to happen to anyone in the family, it was best it was me. I had no children, no husband, no ties.' Judith's view is slightly more positive, but similar feelings of responsibility, this time tinged with shame, emerge: 'I suppose this is character forming for the family, it must have made them more thoughtful. They've all been incredibly good, but I'm just unhappy that it's taking so long. I don't feel it's fair on them.' This inability to control the rate of physical deterioration calls to mind Ricoeur's distinction between flesh and body as the 'primordial form of alterity' (Waldenfels 1996: 116). This difference, at least in part, produced Judith's frustration and Jane's fear of intolerable symptoms or, for others, simply a sense of grim collaboration: 'I can't believe the changes in my body, but I can't help it, can I? If you could stop anything happening you would, but you can't stop anything. There's no control, you can only let it run its course' (Eunice).

As Jane shows, the coalescent effects of physical decline, inhibited personal autonomy and painful feelings of inadequacy can permeate even the most intimate and private of moments: 'You have to give in and have things done for you. Like now, I can't do anything. I even have to be fed and that is very, very hard. I wait as long as possible before going to the loo. It is so embarrassing when you're not in control. You've got to rely on someone else and that's frightening and hard at the same time.' Even Jane's 'good days' were haunted by her dread of uncontrollable symptoms. Not just the common fear of recurrent pain, but the prospect of being unable to breathe or to communicate her distress: 'They say you don't suffocate, but how do they know? If you're laying there in a coma, how do they know you're not suffering?'

Although she was unable to entrust herself to others, Jane was also terrified of being left alone: 'I take as much Lorazepam as I can for the panic. As soon as anyone leaves, I feel panic come over me. It's a horrible feeling.' Such dread is well documented amongst people suffering from motor neurone disease (Barby and Leigh 1995; Holden 1980). It is hard to imagine a more urgent declaration of the existential terror that arises from realizing one's inability to change places with another. Truly, 'existence is the sole thing I cannot communicate, I can tell about it, but I cannot share my existence. Solitude thus appears as the very event of being' (Levinas in Nemo 1985: 57).

If the solution to this situation lies, not in escaping solitude, but in escaping being, then Jane's anxieties and the solution to which she sometimes alluded, suicide, would seem to indicate that our most fundamental or authentic relationship cannot be with another person, but with death. Jane herself, however, undermines this radical isolation. Personhood may not be shared in any sense that dispels its uniqueness, but it can be addressed in ways that make its experience less painful. For Jane, 'at least here in the hospice some of the panic went. I knew someone was here all the time. I wasn't on my own. I only had to touch the button and someone was there.' Comforted by the knowledge that not all communication is verbal or gesticulatory, reassured by the care she received from nurses trained to observe subtle indicators of distress (even in the apparently unconscious patient), Jane sometimes relaxed, finding security because 'they're watching over you all the time'.

Communication: autonomy and authenticity

An inability to express suffering is not confined to those who are paralysed. For many people in this study, their isolation was compounded by feelings of communicative powerlessness, by their inability to raise painful topics and by the reluctance of their family and friends to acknowledge their situation: 'Life isn't very good now. I'm not winning and this is going to kill me in the end. But people don't want you to accept it. They think you're giving in. It puts pressure on me' (Elspeth). When someone is terminally ill, secrecy, ambivalence, indirection and conflict in family communication are not uncommon developments. At least three people in this study were communicating via a third party with friends or relatives whom they previously regarded as special or close. Elspeth, for instance, recognized that by never initiating 'difficult' topics of conversation with her family she was abdicating responsibility, 'giving away' her control and power. She spoke sadly and with resentment of the non-communication between herself and her husband: 'My family all try to ignore what's happening. We don't talk about it. My husband, Bill, is a bit deaf. It might be on purpose. Some people are and then they don't get bothered by the problems of the world.'

Coincidentally, at the end of this conversation, Bill entered her room carrying a clean nightdress in a carrier bag. Elspeth responded sharply 'Oh, it's not what I wanted, and the bag is going to clutter up, it's not what I asked for.' Bill quietly apologized and went to the day room for a smoke. Later, I found him sitting in the corner with his back to the room, crying. Without advocating a brutal transparency, Bill and Elspeth's situation suggests that when significant cues are ignored and real issues are side-stepped, even from an understandable desire to protect, pain may actually be magnified. Insignificant details can become charged and communication fractured and awkward. Repressed or disowned truths do not disappear but can assume maverick and destructive qualities. In this instance, Longaker's (1997: 98) words surely apply to both husband and wife: 'What we fail to realize is that by considering death to be tragic and hopeless we end up making it that way, because we let our fears inhibit us from genuinely connecting and sharing our life and our love. I often tell family members "to be told you are dying is not the worst thing that can happen to you. The worse thing is to feel abandoned in a time of crisis." When we avoid speaking about the coming death, we unknowingly isolate the dying person during the greatest physical and emotional pain of his life. Even if he is surrounded by friends, when they cannot share the truth together, the dying person will feel alone and abandoned.'

Authentic communication involves risk, and risk makes demands of trust. Trust and betrayal, however 'contain each other' (Hillman 1978: 66). Hillman tells a Jewish story that points to an ultimate dimension in all acts of risk. A loving father allows his young son to badly fall when, in one final act of play, the boy jumps from a wall, imagining he will once more safely land in his father's arms. For Hillman, 'The broken promise is a breakthrough of life in the world of Logos security, where the order of everything can be depended upon and the past guarantees the future. The broken promise or broken trust is at the same time a breakthrough to another level of consciousness (Hillman 1978: 65). The father says, in short, I have betrayed you as all are betrayed in the treachery of life created by God. The boy's initiation into life is initiation into adult tragedy' (Hillman 1978: 68).

Similarly, Bill and Elspeth's difficulties implicitly invite them to a deeper level of awareness. It is imperative, therefore, that professionals have sufficient tact and sensitivity to recognize this potential and to offer appropriate support for its realization. If, however, they also communicate without authenticity—talking at, rather than to, patients, not listening, ignoring verbal hints, body language or symbolic suggestions or withholding information—they can compound tragedy. There is always the danger that, in the eyes of the patient, such indirect communication assumes the proportions of a conspiracy, a plot designed to limit their understanding and autonomy, even their chances of survival. To Julia, for instance, 'it seemed important to be in control, not at the mercy of the doctors. I wouldn't be at all surprised if there was some sort of experiment going on, but I wouldn't let the doctors finish me off, even if they had sort of decided it would be kindest to let me die.'

Patients always appreciated clear, honest and sensitive communication, even of painful truths. Many, such as Debbie, felt that to be informed was to be empowered: 'It's about taking control and doing the best you can, because sometimes when you're diagnosed, the hole is there, already dug, just waiting for you to jump in. You can be pushed in slowly too, just because you're not given certain information. I had to fight for a book on chemotherapy, beg for a book on radiotherapy and plead to get the names of drugs and what their side effects would be.' If patients are not given appropriate information, their efforts to retain any self-determination can be exhausting and defensive. As Debbie found, any non-conformity is also likely to result in their being labelled and treated as awkward: 'In hospital I wouldn't take the medication. I was in a circle trying to keep up with what was going on. But it was a case of "We're going to drug you up so you'll lay down in the bed and you're quiet and don't give us any trouble."'

Despite all the disempowering consequences of a terminal illness, patients indisputably make cognitive efforts to manage their psychological stress (Lazarus 1993). Much of what is labelled 'defence' may actually be a 'reconstructive activity' (Ersek 1992; Salander et al. 1996) to this end. The development of protective illusions (as distinct from delusions) where patients compare themselves favourably with other people facing hardships (Taylor 1983, 1989) or the way some even draw inspiration from the deaths of others, may be similarly interpreted. Thus, Mary thought 'a lot about the starving places in Africa and stuff like that' and Judith tried to emulate her heroine, the cellist Jacqueline du Pré, who died tragically young from a paralysing disease: 'She was so talented, so young, when she died. I mean, why her? But it was her and she had to make the best of it too.' In what is a potentially intolerable and uncontrollable situation, however, temporal metaphors are the strategic response, *par excellence*. This again demonstrates that the prism (Fig. 6.1) constructed from metaphors that mediate life for terminally ill people is only encountered adequately when it is considered holistically.

Temporality: agency of control

Generally, it is reference to the natural order and to preoccupation that determines the 'movement' of time, not the thing itself. We may speak of taking time to, having time for, losing time, but all our metaphors and measurements are abstract presentations. How, therefore, can time be 'long' or 'short' when its 'being' is inaccessible to us (Ricoeur 1984: Vol.1, 63)? Nevertheless, these (and others) are the temporal metaphors by which we live. In serious illness, however, their reassuring enclosures are less substantial. Artificial light, strict drug regimens, disturbed patterns of sleep, these may all distort expectation, memory and attention. Naming a fear partially disarms it by establishing parameters. The many efforts patients make to restore what we conventionally take for the 'being' of time is a similar defensive response and demonstrates how effectively encounters with 'non-being' elicit fear, insecurity and sensations of powerlessness. Temporal myopia can be a form of spiritual resistance, a defence against ultimate enquiry whose breach may result in existential distress. To apprehend the non-being of time, to wonder where I, finite being, stand in relation to infinity, is an enquiry very many people—healthy as well as ill, simply find too discomforting to handle.

It is hardly surprising, then, if patients try to 'reconstruct' time by creating new modalities of past, present and future. The latter tends to be either avoided, 'I won't plan ahead' (Debbie), 'There is no future now' (Elsie) or handled in terms of a perpetual present, 'To hell with it, I'm just going to live as though I'm going to live for ever' (Julia). Patients would try to block 'bad signs' or find ways of interpreting them more benignly. Josie's decision to foster a qualitative appreciation of time, for example, both asserts and bolsters her sense of personal autonomy: 'I was worried when I was sick today. Teeth all chattering and out of control. I said to the nurse "Is this the start of the decline?" But I mustn't think that things are a bad sign otherwise my life won't be quality time will it? It'll just be being anxious.'

Despite such efforts, Eileen demonstrates how the dreams of terminally ill people will betray their deeper concerns (Welman and Faber 1992): 'I do think about dying and feel really, really scared. I try to put it at the back of my mind, but it's there all the time. Night time is the worse. I have horrible dreams. I'm in this big white place. Everything is white. I wake myself up, just to prove I'm still here.' Just as trust and betrayal, being and non-being are mutually implicated, perhaps an experienced spiritual director could have helped Eileen to discover a less terrifying 'non-white'. Non-being and loss of control do frighten, but—much as a diver might initially mistake a rescuing dolphin for a shark—our deepest fear may turn out to be our greatest friend. Similarly, the apparently marginal situation may carry a liminal potential. Fear speaks of bravery, absence implies presence and Edinger (1973: 224) convincingly argues that 'dreams suggest an urgency on the part of the unconscious to convey awareness of a metaphysical reality, as if such awareness were important to have before one's death.' Physically isolated and often in pain it is hardly surprising if Eileen felt too vulnerable for such explorations. Her resistance, however, required tremendous energy and she was clearly emotionally depleted, littering her speech with references, if not to death, then to its artefacts: 'They were going to send me for a CAT scan, but I talked them out of that. It reminds me of a coffin. It's the nearest I've been to a coffin. It's all padded. Knowing that I can't move in there, I break into a sweat.' Deriding what she called the 'silliness' of this reason, Eileen told medical staff she did not want the scan because she had 'come to terms' with her diagnosis, a statement rendered transparent by her fearful dream. Although she clearly felt the 'logical' explanation was the more acceptable, her post-interview satisfaction, 'it was lovely, a relief just to talk, beautiful', and her retention of her transcript, suggest less rational unmet needs.

The efforts involved in sustaining temporal myopia take various forms (Charmaz 1983: 241). Each is designed to reassert a sense of control and to keep anxious feelings at bay. Patients might try to adhere themselves to the present by cramming their time with a superficial 'busyness'. Julia provides an ironic example. Preferring to drive than to rest, she felt more 'normal' when she was most a stranger: 'I used to take off in the car. I just went away by myself, to where I wasn't a sick person. I wasn't a cancer patient. I could behave like a normal person.' In her particularly desolate moments, she found relief in a movement and activity which many would consider extraordinary: 'One day I drove around 140 miles. I was absolutely shattered when I got home, but no worse than if I'd just lain there feeling sorry for myself.'

When the future is thought of as a place, travelling can (re)create time frames safer than those scheduled by sickness. Imaginary journeys also foster comforting fantasies, 'you never know what's around the next corner—someone might come up with a wonder drug' (Fred), and 'final' destinations are out-manoeuvred. That is, until some chance phrase or insight jerks the 'escapee' back to what Jane called 'this world'. She would 'lie in bed thinking of holidays. It's an escape route really, but when one of my friends said something, I suddenly thought "I might not be here in a couple of months." It suddenly struck me and I felt frightened.'

Even when very ill, Claude spoke with enthusiasm of returning to Africa. Eventually, he accepted a day trip organized by the day centre as his most realistic option. Again, temporal metaphor and travel are mutually implicated: 'I'm thinking about going to Victoria Falls. I look at our photographs but try not to think about the past, I think it's the future that's important, but I don't really think about the future either. I've been talking to the day centre about bird watching. I'm hoping it might come off, I'm living day to day.' Even when surrounded by glossy holiday brochures, Claude never entirely eclipsed the seriousness of his situation. Once he expressed a wish to be cremated almost in the same breath as planning to visit Africa. This example is crude, but patients often accommodate a quite subtle 'double knowledge' (Weisman 1972). To swiftly apply labels of denial every time a patient makes impossible plans is analogous, perhaps, with dismissing the inherent wisdom of a Zen koan or insoluble conundrum. Where painful topics are concerned, complex paradoxes and tensions are often played out in a mental and emotional choreography of approach and avoidance. Much as Eileen couched her refusal of a CAT scan in logical but transparent terms, the painful tensions between Claude's poor prognosis and his brittle optimism are only just submerged: 'When you write to your friends, they immediately think you are at death's door and visit, so I've been telling them I'm not in pain, I'm only in the Hospice because the staff–patient ratio is so much higher. Although, I suppose, it will probably be the last chance I have to see many of them.' His ambivalent feelings were betrayed by a simple omission. Signing a document usually indicates some concordance with its contents. Intriguingly, Claude 'forgot' to sign these letters. Only an alert recipient realized his identity.

Patients' recurring talk of travel, whether intended literally or metaphorically, calls to mind an ancient symbol of incarnation: the four-wheeled chariot (Luke 1987: 107). Perhaps the vehicular preoccupation of certain patients (for travel always requires some mode, even if it is walking) indicates both their awareness of impending mortality, as much as any yearning for health. Interestingly, Irene, resigned and phlegmatic, compared her situation to being stuck in traffic. Her healthy husband could drive but she could not. 'If my husband gets het up, I say, "It's like we're in this traffic queue. Accept we can't go anywhere and we'll sit here." I say to him "Calm down, or you'll have a heart attack and I can't drive."' Similarly, Elsie associated impotence with images of defective transport: 'It's not worth planning at my age, 82. There's no chance of anything. You can't get on buses or anything. They go before you sit down and you can't control it.'

Destination and destiny, with their connotations of fixture and schedules beyond human control, are etymological cousins. Consequently, when the future is thought of in terms of a series of disembarkation points, a firm prognosis somehow substantiates death, making it an unavoidable event or destination. The repression of tremulous curiosity—lest its expression actually calls its object into being—'roots' patients in the present and may be read as a fearful attempt to 'stop' time, to prevent death. Sadie puts it thus: 'I can't do anything and I don't know what's going to happen. I don't want to ask the doctors, but I don't want to wait and see. I just don't want to move from where I am. I'm such a coward. It's so difficult for me.'

In such a situation, distracting activities are valued not simply for their own sake but because they simulate motion without implying progression. Unsurprisingly, rather than ruining the present by dwelling on 'how long' they might have 'left' or how they might die, many patients simply chose to 'get by, one day at a time' (Eileen). Handled in this manner, the one common certainty, dying, can even acquire a conditional status: 'They didn't give me a time and I don't really want it. If it will happen it will happen' (Irene). In fact, the only attempted prognosis was wildly inaccurate and, months later, still bitterly resented by its recipient, Carla: 'Just before Christmas he gave me three to four weeks. That was the WORST THING [shouted] he could ever have done. He totally ruined our Christmas. If he hadn't said that, I would have had more fight to go through Christmas. He broke my hope. I just hadn't given myself that time limit.'

Some people reduced the traumatic significance of the future by immediately despatching ominous tasks. These were then 'forgotten' or spoken of merely in terms of an insurance policy— just in case. 'I only look to the future in stages. The first thing I did was sort out my will and the care of my son. If anything should happen to me, I won't have to talk about it later on. It was like my spirit was saying, "If you do certain things now, Debbie, it will make it easier later on." And it really has, because I don't have to think about it now.' Fred arranged his finances and Josie spoke with her family about the kind of funeral she would like, even the clothes she wanted to wear. Tracey arranged the legal custody of her children, characteristically protesting 'Just because I know I'm dying, an' get ready, it don't mean I'm jus' gonna lay down and die. I ain't dead yet.' All this sorting calls to mind Berger's (1969) first signal of transcendence—the human propensity to order. Ultimately, this propensity stems from a conviction that, despite all appearances, 'all will be well'. Rather than leading to an attitude of childish irresponsibility or fatalism, it can be liberating to realize that, beyond a certain point, we are not responsible for life. Worrying becomes pointless and 'letting go' of certain anxieties or desires makes sense. Once Gregory's major worry, the future care of his wife, was settled, he was sad to think 'I won't see my family. I won't see my two young grandchildren married with children' but he also concluded 'what I've no control over, what I don't understand, I just try and put in the background.' Similarly, although Josie guessed her son's needs, her reservations about meeting them make sense: 'My son wants to confide in me about something. I'd like to help him, but not totally. I've got to let go of that, because I'll be passed on, and he'll have to carry on with his own life by himself.' Clearly, this is a point at which metaphors of 'control' and 'letting go' coalesce, illustrating that in matters of human experience 'truth' is rarely expressed in formulas of 'either/or' or 'this or that'.

Companionship and absorbing activity may shield patients against the knowledge of impinging mortality but, even when they are too sick to construct these shelters, there is still refuge to be found in reconstructing temporal metaphor. Inevitably, as illness progresses, the pace of life slows down. Charmaz also describes how simple tasks take far longer but the present seems to expand to accommodate them. Where days were once tightly scheduled with a variety of distractions, it is now their drawn-out quality that resists the future. Activity and speed still mediate time but in a manner opposite to cramming life with a relentless activity. The present may come to be characterized more by feelings than by busyness (Charmaz 1983: 243). As Tracey explains, 'You gotta learn to play the time.' For Fred, this meant 'ringing for the nurse, asking for a coffee, even just moving about a bit in the bed. It breaks things up.' Unfortunately, Elsie's inability to control any patterning of her day made her becoming 'rooted in the present' an impossible 'game' to play. 'It's miserable. I'm blind and rely on the district nurse. That means every day you can't plan anything because she never comes at the same time. It's the same with meals on wheels. I was having them at 11 o'clock in the morning, which is daft.' Perhaps as much as physical ability, being able to plan, to choose, to create a personally meaningful temporal structure, makes it possible for terminally ill people to sustain a hopeful, but realistic, attitude (Cutcliff 1995; Herth 1990; Hockley 1993).

Ultimate control

The 'Living will' is a document designed to provide patients with some control over their medical care should they lose the ability to communicate. No one in this study, however, mentioned having considered this option, although a number of people stated they were glad to be dying in a hospice where medical interventions might be less vigorous or intrusive than in a hospital. Three people, however, alluded to a more fundamental choice—either the taking of their own life or a desire for legalized voluntary euthanasia (as euthanasia raises an ethical debate beyond the scope of this book, it is here considered only insofar as it relates to the metaphor of control). Jane argued that many patients contemplate suicide, sharing these thoughts only with one another, definitely not with hospice staff. 'Everyone thinks it. When it's really bad, it's helpful just to know that option is there.'

The validity of Jane's argument is hard to judge. If true, then my identification with St Christopher's may have prevented other patients from sharing suicidal thoughts. Alternatively, it is difficult to gauge the extent to which Jane projected some of her darker moods onto others. Just as patients reclaim feelings of control by making favourable downward comparisons, many also found refuge in emphasizing the universality of their experience and their sense of the collective: 'We all have to be born and we all have to die' (Gregory); 'I'm not the only one' (Elsie); 'We all come into this world on our own, and we all go out on our own' (Camilla).

Eunice equated euthanasia with switching off pain, curiously suggesting that death would somehow 'release' the energy sustaining her existence to take effect elsewhere: 'If there was something available to end your life I'd be for it. I've had my life. I'm 82, let someone else have it.' Carla was the only other interviewee who mentioned taking her own life. Her ambivalence and sense of familial responsibility, however, soon emerged: 'Sometimes I'd like a drug, just to go to sleep and not to wake up. They don't practise euthanasia here do they [sounding alarmed]? I had an aunt with similar problems to me who committed suicide. Once I wondered if I could do the same thing, but it's selfish. Although I would like to be right out of it altogether, it would be even worse for your family.'

By choosing not to stage her own death, Carla shifts the focus from 'control-as-a-manipulation' of circumstances towards a positive concern for her husband and children. Paradoxically, by so doing, she demonstrates features of potency that show how 'power and love are interrelated ... One must have power within oneself in order to love in the first place. ... A person must have something to give in order not to be completely taken over or absorbed as a nonentity. The fallacy of the juxtaposition of love and power comes from our seeing love purely as an emotion and power solely as a force of compulsion. We need to understand them both as ontological, as states of being or processes' (May 1972: 114).

Some appreciation of this paradox is essential if metaphors of 'letting go', the fifth facet of the prismatic symbol, are to be adequately addressed. 'Letting go' also implicates and mediates ontology—the nature of our being. Unlike metaphors of control, however, 'letting go' does not require the reification of conventional temporal metaphor. If anything, 'letting go' affirms just how contingent is our understanding of time. Not withstanding all that has been written here, this awareness sometimes solicits not alarm, but reassurance, occasionally even hopeful anticipation.

Chapter 9

Metaphors of letting go

Introduction

To equate 'letting go' only with subdued passivity or as providing a simple diametric to metaphors of control is a mistaken and superficial analysis. Letting go can be a metaphor with exciting, almost invigorating, qualities. So much so, that although it has little in common with control in terms of manipulation, it has much to do with 'trusting to life' and a sense of ultimate order, a belief or recognition that somehow everything 'comes right' in the end. Josie and Eileen demonstrate both points: 'You shouldn't be reckless, but you've got to take some risks in life. The greatest risk of all is not to take any' (Josie); 'Take every day as it comes. Nobody knows what's around the corner. My youngest one got pregnant while she was still at school. It was touch and go whether she had a termination, but he's a smashing kid and we wouldn't be without him now' (Eileen).

Neither does letting go imply capitulation. Josie makes this distinction: 'I'm calm and accepting. But I haven't given up, thrown in the towel; I'm still hoping the drugs will give me a bit of a run.' Her acceptance is qualitatively different from that voiced in rigid stoicism. It seems to require less effort and the distinction is pronounced as much by general demeanour and body language as by what is actually said. Although he was clearly tense and tapping the arm of his chair, Arthur, for example, sounded every inch the defiant old soldier: 'I've seen five people come and go while I've been in here. Dead. That's what you come in for. I know what I've gotta do, and I will. I'm just waiting now.' One cannot fail to admire Arthur's courage and dogged determination to 'do the job right', but from this perspective, death is an event which crashes over one like an ocean wave. There is also an attitude of grim resistance, of bracing oneself against the inevitable. In no sense is death an experience for which one actively prepares, willingly participates and trustingly embarks. Alternatively, when letting go supplies the root metaphor for terms of acceptance, a liminal awareness is sometimes discernable. Mary provides a striking example: 'I want to die. I'm not close enough to that door. I would like to go though that door. There is a bright, bright world inside and I'll be free from pain and from earthly problems. I very much feel there's this other world. It's vast and we don't have the slightest real inclination of what is available.' Similarly, although Carol found 'it has been so difficult to let go', she spoke calmly of her impending death: 'My hope is that it will lead me into peaceful waters. Sailing on a calm sea. I have expended so much anger in the past and have longed to get rid of it. It seems that this tragedy has taken me on that path at last.'

For most people, however, the inherent insecurity of liminality is too threatening and rarely spoken of in liberating terms. Despite the limitations imposed by fraying conventional temporal metaphor and by advancing disease, patients, like the rest of us, are reluctant to relinquish the tried and tested metaphors of control—even if they no longer successfully mediate their novel experiences. In Hazel's opinion, 'there are people here who ought to let go and they can't, they're hanging on to life.' Of course, living by metaphors of letting go cannot preclude all the pains of dying, but Mary shows how the suffering that results from an inability to acknowledge change might be altered: 'The little ones say things like "Will Daddy get married again? Will we know who it is?" A year ago I would have been desperately upset, but now I think, at least they have a healthy outlook—to the future. I don't need to be there as a hole in their lives, stopping things from ever changing. I feel very much released from their lives.' Paradoxically, perhaps this release stems from Mary actively facing or carrying her suffering. Her difficulties have not been obliterated, but their meaning is transformed by a fiat that betokens possibility over submission. An interesting analogy occurs in Native American folklore. Stolen children, by whispering their plan to one another, lean towards their impending destruction, an open fire. This complicity with danger melts the wax used to blind them, so enabling their escape. Upon their release, indicating that life's destructive element is never entirely banished, the hag responsible for their abduction is not destroyed, but falls into the fire and becomes a cloud of mosquitoes which continues to plague mankind.

In palliative care, distinctions between healing and curing, or inevitable and unnecessary suffering, are not novel (Lunn 1996). Their presentation in terms of letting go (Ainsworth-Smith and Speck 1982; Morrison 1994), where letting go is associated with specific tasks (Clark 1990) or identified as the distinctive mind-set of a certain stage of dying (Reimer *et al.* 1991), is also familiar. This book differs in that it tries to draw attention to the metaphoric nature, not only of these interpretations, but also to the first-order propositions they represent (namely the words and deeds of terminally ill people), emphasizing that such metaphors can powerfully disclose patients' spiritual concerns.

Letting go annunciates theological territory for, as convex is to concave, one releases 'into' as well as 'from'. Just as with the American fable, whenever letting go is mobilized, the question 'What kind of a story are we in?' arises at some level. Certainly patients often felt they were not in full possession of their own 'story' and its reasons. Sighing deeply, Mary continued 'I do feel this whole thing has a purpose. There is a reason why I have cancer and why it had to happen to our family, even though it may not make sense now.' For Eileen a horizon of meaning also existed somewhere beyond her grasp: 'I don't know but I suppose this is all sent for a reason. I do think that … even if I can't see it.'

This need to couch personal narrative in epic or ultimate dimensions reveals the depths of human spiritual yearning, the desire to 'make sense' at the furthest point of existential enquiry. Even the apparently contradictory actions of Jane, self-professed atheist, point in this direction. She derived tremendous consolation from speaking with a medium who provided her with a set of relativising and metaphysical terms of reference. Much as Josie had to let go of the desire to meet all her family's needs, only by relinquishing unrealistic hopes for a cure and by locating her experience within a broader horizon could Jane begin to tolerate her situation: 'I went to see a medium a while back. She said "I'm sorry, I can't tell you you'll get better. The only thing I can say is you've got to accept things." And the more I've gone on and accepted it, the better. She said my friends and loved ones in the spirit world are rallying around to help and that made me feel better too. You think you'll never get used to it when another bit [of the body] goes, but it's weird. The mind sort of takes over and tells you different. You cope, you cope.'

When framed in terms of positive acceptance, letting go seems to mediate a comfort that patients interpret as having origins that incorporate but exceed the near at hand. Furthermore, as symbolized earlier by the indestructible insects, life continually presents opportunities for human beings to realize this metaphor. This realization is not simply 'knowing about' in a cognitive sense, but challenges the whole person. It is a process of becoming. With invigorating imagery, Hazel's reproposition of Pascal's wager reveals painful ontological demands. Recalling Mary, who only 12 months earlier would have been 'desperately upset' if her children spoke of her husband remarrying, Hazel also suggests a perspective into which one 'grows' through incremental adjustment: 'Letting go of your life is something that can be practised, but it's rather like plunging into the sea. It takes courage. It may be marvellous afterwards or we may not know, so we needn't worry. But death is inevitable and to let go of as much as you can, little by little, eases the way into dying. I've given away my clothes and most of my best books by now—but that's just bragging. I know that letting go is one of the special thoughts I need to have all the time now, but then I retract and don't want to part from anything.' Less dramatically and with a focus more on living than dying, Julia makes a similar point, 'the decisions you make around the late twenties actually decide whether you are going to be a good or a bad person. Only little decisions: the extra cigarette, being nasty to someone, taking the biggest cake. Tiny decisions that, in themselves, don't seem important.'

Could Hazel and Julia's continual choosing be what Steindl-Rast (1981: 12) means by spiritual development? He writes 'the turning point of the spiritual life is the moment when time running out is turned into time being fulfilled. Life is something we have to choose. One isn't alive simply vegetating; it is by choosing, making a decision, that you become alive. In every spiritual tradition, life is not something that you automatically have, it is something you must choose, and what makes you choose is the challenge of death—learning to die, not eventually, but here and now.'

Self-identity, temporal metaphor and the paradoxical freedom that may result from letting go interpenetrate—regardless of whether the letting go is of unrealistic ambitions, unsatisfactory relationships, old grudges or material objects. Recalling the changed perspective of the seer, some patients consciously discarded their earlier future-oriented priorities in favour of a more generalised attitude of kindness or generosity. Inevitably, grief or loss are associated with any re-orientation, but as Debbie's response to her brother's carelessness shows, there can also be a sense of relief: 'My brother borrowed my best leather coat—it cost £450. I saved for it when I was a student. Then, the other day, I went to put it on, but it had a massive rip in one sleeve. Once upon a time, I would have stormed to my brother's room, but when I looked at it I thought "alright, I'll leave it there and get it mended. I'll just tell my brother not to wear it in case it gets any worse." That was it, no noise, no argument, just nice and peaceful. That's nice because, at the end of the day, better the coat get ripped than my brother's arm. I just learned to let the coat go.'

Debbie's archaic 'end of the day', once more indicates the extent to which forgiveness is animated by consciousness of human finitude—implying, at some level, an awareness of infinity. Such refocusing, as earlier discussion of the seer suggests, is an expansive movement. Priorities are reordered, conventional perspectives undermined and it seems inconceivable that a leather coat should arouse anger before concern for one's brother. Debbie also regarded learning to let go as a gradual process of adaptation. Impending discussions of the archetypal hero disclose the pain of some of her 'lessons'. Nevertheless, her welcome, albeit occasional, moments of equanimity (when once there had been none) indicate how discovery of one's place in a larger story may result in unanticipated gifts. The broader horizon places the near at hand in a new perspective, so altering its meaning. In effect, Debbie felt 'It's like finding the meaning of life but not exactly knowing what it is. [laughter] That's how it is, I feel like I'm really alive and living. My spirit is at peace. I don't shout any more. Everything is so smooth now. I've a much better relationship with my son since I became ill. We talk more. Everything is based around life or relates to life and being alive and living. Before that, I was just on a treadmill.'

Renunciation is usually thought of in terms of denial. Debbie, Mary, Josie, Hazel and others, however, suggest that it may be envisaged more generously, as a 'saying yes' (Saunders 1986) to whatever life brings. Just as 'the world is dreadful and fascinating to the child, sexuality is so to the youth, death is so to the man and spirit itself is ultimately so. When one consents to the unknown, however, it seems to lose its dread and fascination, to lose its divinity and become human. The world becomes familiar; sexuality becomes one's manhood or womanhood, death becomes one's mortality and spirit becomes one's self. The difficulty of consenting, though, is that one cannot bring oneself to say yes to the unknown until it seems human, but it does not seem human until one says yes (Dunne 1975: 80).

Beheld in the light of Dunne's words, it is hardly surprising if, after distributing her books, Hazel longed to 'retract', to gather them back. As she remarked, 'It can be frightening to feel that you're shrinking.' Nevertheless, without underestimating any accompanying grief and pain, a generalized affirmation does sometimes resonate in specific actions such as Hazel distributing her books, Fred writing his will or Sadie giving her rings away. Even Irene, whose grim stoicism has already been commented upon, brightened as she recounted joking with her family: 'You say, "do you want this when I've gone?" "No we don't want that!" Or my daughter will say, "What I do want is …" and I say, "Well, you'll have to wait until your dad goes for that, it's part of a set."' Alternatively, Josie found 'Me son, keeps asking if he can have me stereo. I'm not dead yet, but it's like they're going around putting their names on me things and I don't like it.'

Clearly, letting go—like realizing the potential of the limen—is a process that may not be forced. When metaphors of release and holding on compete, pain and internal conflict invariably result. For instance, commenting on the death of a fellow motor neurone disease sufferer, Jane remarked 'He had no quality of life, but when he died I was so angry with him for going off and leaving me. How dare he leave me? I was being selfish because he'd had enough and he told me so. But, oh, I was holding on to him. Of course now, I realize how he felt.'

Hazel framed a similar disengagement more emphatically as 'letting go', rather than as 'not holding on'. The consequences, she felt, were also more likely to be positive: 'I am trying not to demand that my nephew comes to see me every week, which I would like, but he is very busy. You can only have a good relationship if it has the letting go in it. You can't have a good relationship if you are hanging on to that person's company. Not having any children helps me; most people can't let go, so they hang on.' Collaboration with the inevitable has proven helpful in other apparently hopeless situations, so perhaps it is less than surprising if it should appear so to terminally ill people. Non-resistance, for example, characterizes the liberating yoga and meditation sometimes taught in high-security jails. These practices are presented as a form of non-denominational but distinctly spiritual development. It is in the nature of metaphors of letting go and of liminality to intimate accession to another order, to mediate nascent spiritual awareness and so change the 'feel' of immediate circumstances and one's attitude towards them. Late in her illness, for example, when she reflected on an unfair disciplinary hearing at work, Julia found that 'It became trivial, so I actually forgave everybody. All the energy you tie up in old wrongs, sorrows and grief, is like carrying, no, dragging around rotten carcasses attached to your shoulders wherever you go. The thing to do, is to cut them one by one. Look at them, examine them, think "I don't need this" and cut the strings.'

Read psychologically, here is a movement towards a new self-appreciation and sociologically, an expression of social adaptation. There are, however other, perhaps more penetrative insights to be made. Julia's words are remarkably similar to a gruesome passage in Homer's *Iliad*. To revenge the slaying of his friend Patroklus, Achilleus kills Hector and then, appalling many witnesses, drags the body back and forth behind his chariot at the end of the athletic games. This incident is often interpreted as a classical expression of liminality, heralding the imminent arrival of a new era (Stein 1983: 10).

Less striking in its expression, but still concerned with releasing 'dead' material, Carla makes the transitional element explicit: 'I've had to do a lot of making up with people, my sister ... you can't leave earth with a grudge can you? It's not right.' Similarly, Camilla found it became necessary to accept of certain friends 'those who fall by the wayside, they fall by the wayside.' At its deepest point, however, the consent implied in letting go is not about something 'other', but about oneself. Hazel shows how, without necessarily excluding anxieties and fear, metaphors of letting go can disclose ultimate meaning and purpose. Chuckling at her own reflections, she said 'Although I apply letting go to the things I have collected, really, it is important to let go of yourself, so your love can flow out to other people and towards God. Naturally, there is still more than a slight anxiety at the thought of having to die! I'm not convinced our personalities carry on, very likely they shan't. When I think about it, I fall into dangerous cracks and crevices, from time to time.' Interestingly, it is at the limen or threshold that familiar ground is no longer underfoot. Unlike the margin, however, where 'dangerous cracks and crevices' also abound, the limen has a potential to foster healing, as a possibility distinct from curing. It may be rare but by divesting themselves of all that gets in the way, notwithstanding their physical frailties, individuals do sometimes realize a wholeness that includes a spiritual or ultimately significant dimension.

Palliative care literature contains many instances of patient behaviour and experience similar to the examples provided in this book. These instances have generated tremendous discourse on psychological adjustment, managing physical symptoms, dealing with 'unfinished business' or the expression of anthropological rites of passage—amongst many other things. These various approaches, however, are not exhaustive. Certainly, human experience is biological, psychological and social, but not entirely so on any count. After any interpretation, some 'surplus of meaning' always remains (Ricoeur 1976). Hazel's understanding of letting go, which is a theological analysis, draws attention to a dimension of human existence whose validity can only be judged in terms of critical realism, that is, by the capacity of thoughts not dissimilar from her own and from diverse cultures, to survive for centuries. These thoughts still meaningfully 'pattern' human experience and have sustained untold numbers. *The cloud of unknowing*, written by an unknown fourteenth-century mystic (Chopra 1997: 196), bears direct comparison with some of Hazel's comments. He too advises one to

> Let go of this everywhere and this something,
> In exchange for this nowhere and this nothing. Do not
> worry if your sense cannot understand this nothing
> for this is why I love it the better … who is it that
> calls it nothing? Surely it is our outer man and not
> our inner man. Our inner man calls it All.

Similarly, in the *Tibetan book of the dead* is written 'I will abandon all grasping all grasping, yearning and attachment' (Rinpoche 1992: 241). To those who might regard such reflections as esoteric, tangential to modern palliative care, Hazel offers a firm riposte. When I asked 'What most helps you to let go of yourself?', she responded 'A nice environment, clean and cheerful, the nurses and my talks with the chaplain. Being able to stay here as long as I need, not having to be uprooted—and I'm not suffering a lot of pain.' By definition, good palliative care is holistic. For the terminally ill person, all that Hazel cites can contribute to the healing of spiritual pain and restore meaning to life by creating a safe place to be. Whether patients interpret their lives in terms of marginality or liminality it should not be forgotten that all 'boundary situations are ambivalent: they offer potential for creativity, and they threaten disintegration. To remain securely and creatively on the boundary, in the gap, we need to be contained. Walls can be imprisoning, but they can free us up to be that more vulnerable or chaotic' (Ward and Wild 1996: 105).

Obstacles

Even after diagnoses are accepted, reconciliations have been made, last wills and testaments have been drawn up and all manner of 'unfinished business' has been despatched, the ontological challenges and shifts of perspective required by letting go cannot be rushed—either by patients or their relatives: 'I haven't got to the stage yet where I want to die. I might reach a point where enough is enough, but I don't feel that yet' (Camilla). If Jane's husband withdrew to the lavatory whenever a homecare nurse arrived, Tracey sighed 'My husband blanks it totally. Can't accept it at all, won't speak about it. That makes it harder for me, but if they can't accept it, you can't force them.'

Such discrepancies could be the source of anguish and anger, sometimes provoking opposition where love and understanding were most needed. Carla, for instance, reflected on her decision to refuse active treatment: 'I've had enough, I just can't go through that again, but my husband can be difficult. He is such a loving man, but he wants me to take all the drugs. He just won't let go. He doesn't want to. He said he wished he was me. He'd rather be the one dying.' Irene had to be equally assertive with her daughter: 'My youngest one was a bit put out. She thought I should go for the treatment. I said to her [voice raising], "Look, it's not your body, it's mine."'

Accounts of exhausted and perplexed patients, afraid but frustrated, anxious to die yet unable to do so, read as classically liminal. Patients such as Mary and Carla, feeling neither here nor there occupy a wilderness somewhere 'between un-being and being' (Eliot 1944: 18). Any resolution of their Augustinian 'Not yet', however, has to be *con summa* for, as Carla illustrates, the critical shift may not be initiated or made by the will alone: 'I don't know how you let go. Part of me wants to, part doesn't. When I fall asleep I jerk awake. I want to let go, but when I'm asleep I jerk back to consciousness. I try to relax, but I can't make anything happen. If I could just make that jump I'd go.' Mary experienced similar tensions and feelings of disunity: 'My conscious knows that I am going to die. It is really sensible about the fact, but my subconscious doesn't seem to understand this. Every time I try to go to sleep, I jerk awake—even with medication. My subconscious doesn't seem to want to let me go. I presume it's frightened, but my conscious accepts, so it's kind of difficult.'

For one such as Mary, longing to pass through her 'golden door', all that remains is to wait. Hers, however, is not the stance of the stoic old soldier, of the deliberately distracted or of the temporally myopic, it is of another order belonging 'to the agony of death and birth' (Eliot 1944: 24):

> I said to my soul be still, and wait without hope
> For hope would be hope of the wrong thing; wait without love
> For love would be love of the wrong thing; there is yet faith
> But the faith and the love and the hope are all in the waiting.

This kind of patience has long been recognized in theological discourse and Weil (1977: 58) writes 'We do not obtain the most precious gifts by going in search of them but by waiting for them. Man cannot discover them by his own powers and if he sets out to seek for them he will find in their place counterfeits of which he will be unable to discern the falsity.' Perhaps with greater bite, given the topic's intense relevance, Hazel expresses something very similar: 'I have always been on the spiritual quest, but I muddled it all up, going from sculpture to Buddhist meditation and not doing anything solidly. There is still time for God to take me under his wing, and for me to know that, but whether it will happen or not, I can't tell. I persevere, rather incompletely, inadequately. But I know what I long for, what I care about … [voice fading into silence].'

Although such waiting may capitulate before despair or distraction, while it continues it expresses a profound hope and spiritual yearning that does not require a religious language to find expression. Paradoxically, when change does occur, when letting go does realize a liminal potential, it is 'the pivotal moment which has no movement of itself, that permits movement to take place' (Ward and Wild 1996: 48).

Expression as realization

Carla painted primarily not for distraction, but to connect with what she regarded as 'really important'. Two of her pictures (Figs 9.1 and 9.2) provide a tender and moving expression of that 'still movement' associated with a fulcrum.

Persuasively tranquil, both works feature a woman engrossed in her sewing. A delicate floral motif emphasizes the peaceful nature of the two scenes, evoking those 'lilies of the valley that neither reap nor toil' (*Luke* Chapter 12, Verse 27). The women's eyes are closed in an enigmatic but apparently serene introspection and each piece is instantly recognizable as a private 'moment out of time', such as occur in all lives. Generally received with surprise and gratitude, moments such as these (as opposed to the 'endless' split second just before an accident), tend to be characterized by contentment and a certain depth of fulfilment. At any second, either woman could look up, engage the viewer and so transform her exclusive reality, for each is poised where conventional temporal metaphor no longer operates, but is easily re-asserted. Even so, each

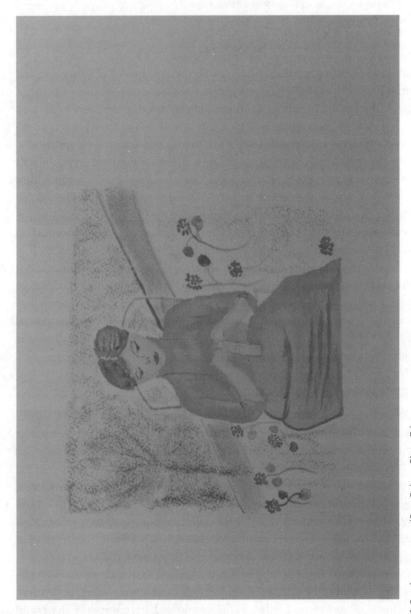

Figure 9.1 Sewing woman. (See Colour Plate 5.)

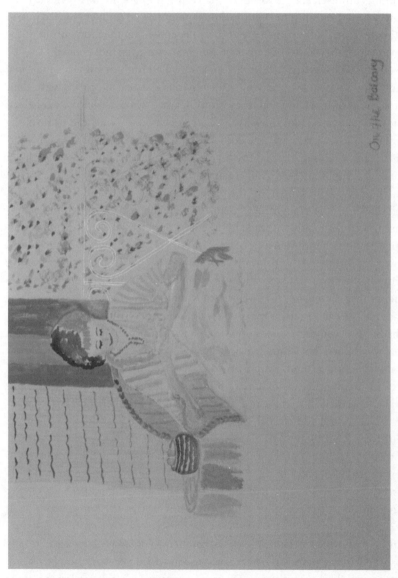

Figure 9.2 On the balcony. (See Colour Plate 6.)

image has a quality of timelessness, suggesting a moment hinged where awareness of finite and infinite coalesce. This pivotal quality finds expression in the balanced symmetrical tension of the balcony railing in Fig. 9.2. In neither painting, however, are the women's feet visible; they are not mistresses of their own destiny. Conventional temporal metaphor may be easily reasserted but, in ultimate terms, both women are entirely dependent on the momentum of the limen which they have entered. Such moments are given, not created.

On the Balcony, title of Fig. 9.7, makes explicit both its subject's marginal and liminal status. Even leaving aside obvious classical allegories, with their intimations of mortality and its evasion (Ariadne whose skein of wool helped Theseus to escape from the labyrinth, or Penelope weaving and unravelling her father-in-law's shroud), the domestic tenderness of these paintings heightens the piercing fragility and mystery of such moments. Indeed, we speak of them as being 'shattered'. This insubstantiality is alluded to by the way in which both pictures 'float' on the paper. The blank surround both contains and challenges the thoughtful women, bringing to mind the difficulties of sustaining a contemplative attitude in the midst of potential engulfment, of realizing the spiritual dimension of contemporary experience. Neither image, however, could exist without practical media—paper, paint, crayons. We glimpse, therefore, not something separate from our material circumstances but another dimension that we generally tend to overlook. If we completely understood each picture, perhaps we would know what happens next—whether the women rise, smile, put down their work. But how can there be a final word when the comprehension illustrated, indeed required, by such work is about letting go and not possession? 'We live in a world of unreality and dreams. To give up our imaginary position as the centre, to renounce it, not only intellectually but in the imaginative part of our soul, that means to awaken to what is real and eternal, to see the true light and hear the true silence. A transformation then takes place at the very roots of our sensibility, in our immediate reception of sense impressions. It is a transformation analogous to that which takes place in the dusk of evening on a road, where we suddenly discern as a tree what we had at first seen as a stooping man ... we see the same colours, we hear the same wind, but not in the same way' (Weil 1977: 93).

It is small wonder that Carla described herself as 'completely lost', 'totally absorbed' in her painting. There is a sense in which her works are prayerful, for through their execution she felt she experienced what she called the 'really real, what really matters'. If needle and thread were replaced by paper and brush, these two works could pass for self-portrait. Losing herself in her work, Carla seemed to acquire—albeit temporarily—many of the qualities she portrayed: 'I never think of smoking when I paint, but normally I chain smoke.' She let go even of her desire 'to make that jump' and, paradoxically, both margin and limen became temporarily habitable.

When metaphors of letting go mediate reality for terminally ill people, their consideration inevitably leads to issues of ultimate as well as human concern. The interests of both carers and theologians are rooted in the same soil of human experience. Although fewer patients in this study reflected upon letting go as a conscious dynamic than were preoccupied with strategies of control, this book is not concerned with statistical representations. Our purpose is to discern spiritually significant patterns of meaning and patients' perceptions of selfhood. Letting go clearly contributes on both counts. Hopefully, a deeper appreciation of this metaphor will awaken sensitivities appropriate, if not to Hermes 'guide of souls', at least to loving and capable companions of people who are terminally ill. Hermes, however, is still a useful point of reference, directing attention to the disclosive potential of archetypal figures generally. This raises at least two questions: do such figures ever mediate patients' experiences and what do they reveal of their spiritual needs? The more I listened to patients, the harder I found it to avoid the archetypal hero, mother and stranger. In an attempt to provide some answers they form the next three facets of the prism.

Chapter 10

Archetypal hero

Introduction

Following much careful listening and observation of terminally ill people, I have presented certain metaphors that seem to mediate their experiences in the form of a symbolic prism (Fig. 6.1). The following discussions of facets six, seven and eight of this prism respectively deal with the archetypal figures of the hero, mother and stranger. Recalling earlier discussions of the significance of archetypes in Chapter 2, these figures emerge both as a product of the psyche but also as a linguistic phenomenon involving archetypal metaphors. Although these metaphors certainly extend to psychological horizons, the following discussions also suggest a disclosive capacity of a further reaching nature.

Despite certain notable exceptions (Kearney 1996; Wheelwright 1981), the potential of archetypal figures to illuminate the experience of terminal illness tends to be approached in terms of maintaining a 'narrative' of the self or of appropriating a socially approved 'media script' such as that of the 'fighting spirit' (Seale 1995). Nearly all authors baulk at the fundamental issue of the origins of archetypal potency. From a perspective concerned with ultimate meaning and purpose, however, the critical question is whether figures such as the archetypal hero, mother or stranger disclose anything of human spiritual needs or awareness. Jung locates the origins of the archetypes firmly within the psyche, both collective and individual, but he also accepts the impossibility of defining the ultimate character of psychic experience (1938: 100). He thus remains open to the possibility of life possessing a dimension of meaning or source that exceeds the creative potential of either the individual or the collective. By deliberately excluding theological discussions from their accounts of human experience, however, contemporary psychology and sociology risk becoming 'closed' intellectual systems. No matter how rigorous a discipline may be, however, there is none which provides an exhaustive explanation of phenomena or whose own perspective is not also a distortion. Even if we are left more questioning than satisfied, research should draw attention to aspects of reality that tend to be overlooked and this is what facets six, seven and eight of the symbolic prism try to do. They make the case for a theological reading of archetypal figures—for their potential to carry ultimate meaning—that is at least as plausible as many psychological or sociological interpretations.

Myth and folklore emphasize the archetypal hero's youth, courage and commitment to his purpose, suggesting that a 'heroic death' may not be universally appropriated. The heroic script, for example, does not fit easily with sudden deaths or in cases such as Alzheimer's disease where the individual may seem to 'disappear' before their actual demise (Seale 1995: 608). The average age of patients whose interview transcripts contained most heroic motifs and metaphors was 44 years and 6 months, whereas the average age for all the participants was 59. From a Jungian perspective this relative youth is unsurprising for the heroic traverse always narrates processes of maturation. Interestingly, long before becoming ill, many of these younger patients framed their life in terms of struggle. Difficult episodes with employers, neighbours, family and friends were often recounted as a relevant prelude to their current battles with cancer. By interpreting their illness as a goal to dwarf all others, these patients experienced the security of a clear sense of purpose and meaning. Julia, for example, 'was really pleased to switch from anger with the housing department, which was like fighting fog, to fighting cancer, which was a nice, clean, straightforward fight. I knew what had to do. I was determined to get back at those people by surviving, to get my revenge, because I was so unfairly treated. I wanted to make that anger positive.'

Traditionally of humble origin, the hero's potential is initially unrecognized—even by himself. It is the unfolding of his destiny, mediated by metaphors of journey and hazard that reveals his abilities and maximizes his identity. Nevertheless, there is always a decisive point at which he takes up his quest and shapes his strategy. Once the fundamental decision is made, self-discipline, courage, independence and strategy tend to be emphasized, along with their astonishing consequences: 'Looking back, if somebody had turned round and said "You'll get cancer next year", I would have thought "Cor, No!" I couldn't have handled it. I'd have topped meself. The following year comes along and I have got cancer but it's "How do we fight it?" I didn't think I could fight it like I have, but somehow I have, and it's made a big difference because it's added a discipline to my life, or rather kept a discipline' (Fred). Tracey was similarly proud of her efforts and achievements, 'Yeah, I've done well to still be here, I'm pleased with meself.'

Modern applications of the heroic narrative, however, tend to overlook its frequent apotheosis: the necessary death of the hero in recompense for hubris or over-reaching pride. Alternatively, he is betrayed or offers himself as a sacrifice that portends a 'new day' for others. Jane's concern shows how metaphors of 'letting go' and heroism can inter-relate. She clearly felt letting go was the braver option; 'When it's my turn to go, will I fight to stay? At the moment I think I've had enough, but what if natural instincts to fight take over? I'm a bit worried about that, because the longer you fight, the longer you hang around. I don't think that's fair on the relatives. They know that you're fighting to hang on to that last little breath. It's a lot easier for them if you let go.'

Palliative literature is divided concerning the significance of the heroic response. While there is some evidence that a 'fighting spirit' not only improves quality of life and perhaps also its quantity, for others it simply betokens an exhausting and potentially harmful struggle. Seale (1995) is unusual in framing the 'struggle to know medical truths', the 'strain of knowing' and finally, the 'acceptance of death' in heroic rather than purely sequential terms. His argument that patients relieve the suffering of others by adopting a heroic stance raises an important question. Just how far does this archetype actually serve patients and their families? For Jane, super-human efforts no longer seemed worthwhile: 'Without my collar on, my head drops forwards and it's a hell of a job to get it back up again. My throat pressing down tends to stop me breathing and I'm frightened. It's all fight, fight, fight. By the end of the day, it's lovely to have a rest from it.' In Julia's case especially, her single-minded pursuit of health called down many dangers associated with the hubristic hero: exhaustion, isolation and the fear of failure.

Popularly, the heroic response equates only with all-out combat and reads more as a caricature than an accurate depiction of complex and subtle thoughts and feelings. It is too simple to regard the heroic archetype simply as a denial of mortality. Awareness is a fluctuating attribute and, as Tracey demonstrates, attempts to out-manoeuvre death do not necessarily deny its inevitability: 'I'll always fight it. I know it will beat me in the end but I won't just give up and die—it won't get me that easy.' Something of the notion of 'right times' and 'wrong times' resonates here—the inevitable is accepted, but it is also recognized that one shouldn't start dying 'too early'. The heroism lies less in rejecting death than in embracing life. The two responses, however, are not simple opposites and distinguishing between short-term (realistic) and long-term (false) hopes is useful here, for patients simultaneously inhabit both temporal realms. All but two patients whose experiences were mediated by the heroic archetype (one of whom was Julia), acknowledged their foresee-able demise. Paradoxically, it appears that death can be simultaneously fought, yet accepted.

Identity security and purpose

The archetypal hero offers security and identity, perhaps because he has specific tasks to accomplish, trials to overcome or enemies within and without to vanquish. In myth or folklore, his challenges are partly 'tamed' by their highly concrete terms: separating wheat from chaff, felling a forest overnight, solving an apparently impossible riddle. The hero's strategies vary and in fairy tales he sometimes derives help from unexpected sources such as a withered crone, a little bird or a talking animal. There is also a sense in which his tasks are non-transferable. Fred, for example, spoke of 'breaking up' his depression. No one else could do this for him and he emphasized the making of finely tuned judgements: 'It's about constantly making choices. I knew I should have the energy either for a bath or a walk today, so I chose the walk.' Specific aims and objectives endow the hero's journey with its characteristic momentum and purpose. Julia also proudly noted her victorious landmarks: 'I can go up the stairs without collapsing which I couldn't 6 weeks ago. I can stay over at friends until half-past one, which I couldn't after my chemo.'

In serious illness, small achievements can be extremely meaningful. For Debbie, 'All the struggles, all the uphill climbs, they have all helped to make me that bit stronger.' The heroic narrative can also accommodate goals less daunting than a full recovery. Purposeful and realistic struggles can energize, build confidence and make life more satisfying: 'My next goal is to walk about 10 yards, and then to the end of the corridor. You've got to hang on and be positive. You enjoy your life a lot more' (Fred). Incremental goals distract from the terminal aspects of disease, without necessarily requiring its denial. Carla found that when she was 'having the hip operation and the traction, I forgot about the cancer. I actually forgot about it. Really forgot about it. I was just concerned that I wanted to walk. That was all that was on my mind—until recently.' Sadly, she discovered that the teleological impulse expended in surmounting a series of obstacles, can also lead to feelings of deflation and disorientation: 'Now that my hip's recovering, there is nothing left to strive for. I know there's the cancer, but it's as if there's nothing left that I can fight. It's as if I'm left high and dry.'

There is no disputing the perseverance associated with heroic identification and exhaustion and collapse are real possibilities. When faced by the patient who is 'doing so well' or 'trying so hard', carers should be alert to such risks. Their need for support may be sudden and urgent, especially if they have commenced a specific 'task': 'Even with the cancer, I managed to build a kitchen from nothing. I may have been hobbling around on me sticks doing 20 minutes work to an hour's rest, but it gave me tremendous satisfaction. I was determined I'd drain the last drop of energy before I'd give in and fall into the reclining chair' (Fred). Clearly, as a complex mediator of events, the heroic archetype is not without its dangers.

Potential snares

Psychological readings of fairy tales (Bettelheim 1991) suggest that to preserve his own infallibility, the hero tends to project his undesirable attributes on to others in a process known as splitting. Julia may have experienced her encounters with the medical profession as 'doctors wanting to "infantilize" me', but her world view was confrontational long before she became ill. Various colleagues were often described as 'bastards'. Considering Julia's portrait, both of herself and her employment situation, there is something almost inevitable about her heroic identification as a patient: 'I was in the most racist part of the borough with an ideal, a crusade to follow. I am an incredibly obstinate ex-Catholic. Also, as a manager, women at work would come to me because there was so much low-grade sexual harassment.' In the hero's eyes, his 'crusade' is inviolate and this distinguishes him from 'ordinary' people. Furthermore his unrealistic self-expectations prevent him from witnessing, let alone sharing, his own portion of the unbearable 'common lot': 'Other people are expected to get thinner and weaker, but I'm the exception. I shouldn't even be in a hospice' announced a quite emaciated Julia.

Just as it is impossible to distinguish marginal from liminal experiences according to their external circumstances, detection of an archetypal presence is no predictor of its consequences. Julia was remorselessly driven, speaking in terms of 'crusade', 'revenge', 'bastards' and confrontation—sometimes when people were actually trying to help her. For instance, 'The doctor said, "What do you mean, you don't feel well?" And I remember thinking, this is no time for a bloody interrogation.' Alternatively, Fred was popular, easy going. The way he dealt with his challenges contributed to the quality of his life. Julia, despite claiming to cherish her body, required at least two emergency respite admissions.

Positive thought is a mainstay of the cancer hero's armamentarium, but the hero's journey is often lonely, through foreign territories and alienated from the near at hand. Julia's frustration perhaps expresses as much about her own dislocated existence, as that of her mother. As experience, maturity and summoning caution are derided, Icarus' ungrounded optimism is summarized and his fate—falling from the sky as his waxen wings melted, is surely portended: 'I'm eternally optimistic, very positive. I won't accept any negative reactions. But every time I telephone my mother, it's either too wet or too cold, too bright or too dark. How can she live like this, in a world she's never at rights with?' (Julia).

When the hero admits his negativity, his fractured perfection, he feels endangered. The diabolic function is to divide: 'I'm angry, and it comes out ... like the devil ... a bad part of me' (Claire) and it is the hero's desire for health, for a wholeness too narrowly defined, that may render him not only one dimensional but also vulnerable. By rejecting what he regards as 'negative' feelings, his emotional range and sensitivity are restricted. If only the consistently positive is acceptable, not only may 'quirky' opportunities be disregarded but, like a table balancing on three perfect legs instead of four uneven ones, very little provocation can result in disaster. Perfection is a finished product, but the hero is identified as much by his journey as his arrival. His is a story of personal development requiring an attitude of flexibility, a willingness to change and the courage to 'let go' of many previous held assumptions.

There is a dangerous trap waiting for those who reify only the hero triumphant and ignore these other aspects of his journey or character. One cannot help but wonder whether Julia became ensnared. The stasis of perfection not only opposes the teleology of the narrative form from which the hero arises, but contradicts processes that accommodate vulnerability, failure and imperfection. Accepting these weaknesses can open up escape routes from a striving isolation, allowing individuals to seek and to accept suitable help. Explaining why she sometimes avoided health professionals, Julia illustrates the lonely antithesis: 'I will never allow getting worse to become a real possibility. At St Christopher's, there's too much acceptance of death. People are expected to die, and lots of us don't [voice fading], not for years and years and years.'

Approval: benefits and costs

Despite any risks involved, attempts to realize the heroic ideal nevertheless carry a high degree of social approval (Gray and Doan 1990). They affirm the masculine ideal, assure a positive reputation after death, help family and friends to cope and can be a source of positive self-esteem: 'All the chaps at work, all of them have said, "Oh, how brave you are." I try to make the best of it, and that makes it easier for them to handle' (Fred), while Carla preened whenever she remembered how her doctor described her as, "a fighter".

A patient's heroic response to cancer not only elicits admiration but can veil a dangerous seduction—ripe both for disreputable exploitation and unconscious enactment. Gray and Doan (1990: 38) ask 'Who amongst us isn't grateful for the opportunity to support a patient's courage and fighting spirit?'

They point to the ease with which a professional may undermine the team ethos of modern palliative care by unwittingly, or otherwise, assuming the mantle of guru or strong tutelary figure: 'The danger is that when practitioners adopt the role of Hero's guide, the patient's visit can become a battleground for reassuring the practitioner about his/her personal power and ability to manage grief and despair' (Gray and Doan 1990: 38).

Sick people are highly vulnerable to powerful forces of transference and to disreputable suggestion. Some weeks prior to her admission to St Christopher's, Claire had disastrously discontinued all her medication on the advice of a faith healer. Later, even as she acknowledged his criminal record and lay desperately ill, she still idealized this man: 'He's very nice. None of this is his fault. I mean, he's been to prison, he's got a history but he is a wonderful man. He does laying on of hands, but maybe you've just got to do it all for yourself [whispering] … with no other people.' It is fear that lies at the base of this faith. Jung (1996: 106) argues that any idealizing of another is a hidden form of turning away (apotropaism) that indicates a deep need to drive away a secret fear. Furthermore, because the hero may not delegate his trials but must, as Claire says 'do it all himself', any disappointments can only signify his own inadequacies. Shared by Debbie, this attitude of total self-reliance—'I have to be independent, I have to keep myself going, no matter what'—can result not only in a highly judgemental view of self but also of others, of their efforts and what they 'merit'. 'Some people, you just know they don't want to be well, not enough. My friend wouldn't give up smoking, so when we went to a faith healer she was really hoping for a miracle. But miracles happen because you are there and ready. You've done all the preparation, they don't just descend' (Julia).

Following Jung, if identification with the hero is about the adventures of personal development, then just as the whale swallowed Jonah, moments of fearful submission or apparent failure may be necessary to the whole process. More typically, however, the heroic archetype manifests in a resistance that sometimes makes things worse. Julia's desperate motoring 'to be somewhere where I was normal', for example, undoubtedly contributed to her exhausted need for emergency respite care. Even if patients do want to 'let go', family and friends may insist they continue to fight. Feelings of shame, personal disappointment, even anger, may stem from any 'failure' to match the ideal. If someone as resolute and strong willed as Julia experienced such pressures, one can only wonder at how much greater they may have been for other patients: 'I hated everyone ringing me up and asking me how I was. Actually they were asking for reassurance, so if I didn't say I felt better, or just said I felt bad, they made me feel guilty for disappointing them.'

Rebel or ally?

One of Julia's respite admissions coincided with my weeks as participant observer and it was interesting to witness the heroic archetype 'in action', as it were. Julia followed a low-fat vegetarian diet but, for the first 3 days of her stay, her meals were unsuitable. Eventually, the senior chef came to see her, requesting she provide him with specific recipes. Julia seemed to interpret these difficulties in two ways, using them to distinguish herself from other patients (the hero is unique) but also to reaffirm her conspiratorial and threatening world view (the hero is rarely 'at home'): 'I think the culture at St Christopher's is most surprising. For people to go in and get weaker is actually acceptable. It's the norm. Nobody picked up on the fact it was wrong for me. I was expected to deteriorate by everybody apart from me. Nobody took on the fact I was not getting enough food to help my recovery. I was the peculiarity.'

Julia's meeting with the chef was the latest denouement in a constant vendetta between ward and kitchen. It allowed the nurses to unconsciously, and sometimes knowingly, champion Julia's cause in such a way that her complaint voiced their more generalized culinary frustrations. By so doing, she made their points whilst they maintained the acceptably composed face of the carer. Confrontation does not sit easily in the hospice ethos of 'niceness' (Speck 1994) and Julia hinted that ownership of this struggle was inappropriately delegated: 'The nurses fought for me and the doctor was upset, but it was left to me to fight, but I wasn't well enough. I couldn't fight.'

Julia revealed, in this and other instances, that she felt manipulated. It was not novel for her to find herself the object of what Buber (1958) calls an 'I–It' relationship. Here she remarks of one hospital admission, 'Doctor X put me on Y ward because he wanted me to stir up the doctors and the nurses. He thought it might do them some good, especially some of the younger ones.' Enlisting patients in the education of junior professionals or to articulate the shortcomings of an institution, is sometimes wise. Only, however, if recruiters are conscious of their own motivation and patients understand and are willing about what is happening. They may inspire, but 'heroes' can also seem 'difficult' patients—determined, distrustful, with a blinkered outlook. Carers may be tempted to recruit their energies 'more appropriately' but it should never be forgotten that the hero is invariably wounded in his traverse. His courage exacts costs and it is inexcusable to use him to reach ends that are not his own or to persuade him along a route not of his own choosing. It is important to ask whether the patient is being empowered or whether patronizing, diversionary and silencing tactics are operational. It may even be the case that any desire to 'win over' such a patient expresses carers' own needs for emotional protection. Making the 'awkward pupil' the 'head prefect' is famous as a castration of equality and a diffusion of real issues. The imperative never to forget exactly whose points are being made is a powerful argument in favour of the discursive forum provided by an interdisciplinary care team.

The scarred hero

Physical alteration, as every warrior knows, can indicate past experiences, future hopes and inner determination. In an interesting inversion of Samson's story, 'many women instinctively cut their hair when they need to be strong' (Bolen 1996: 159). Recalling earlier discussions of control and interpenetrating metaphors, Debbie cut her hair 'because it was more painful to wake up and see it on the pillow than to take control and cut it all off. That was something simple that really helped me. I told the other people I met at chemotherapy and one woman with beautiful red hair down to her waist, had it neck length the following week. She took control.'

At one level Debbie's action was clearly liberating but, at another, her 'Joan of Arc' singularity, extreme independence and self-sufficiency increased her vulnerability. Eventually, because she felt her husband's pain excessively depleted her own emotional resources, Debbie found herself pitted against her potentially most valuable ally: 'I was going to the hospital on my own and my husband hated that. He wanted to be there to support me. Looking back, I could have made it easier for both of us if I had allowed him. But I needed to keep a distance. He would cry, which would cause me to cry. Then, whenever I got home, there were 101 questions, most I had already asked the medical staff but they couldn't answer. He didn't believe me, he thought I was lying ... it just got ... I felt that I needed some space, so I asked him to leave [voice fading]. I ended by hitting him with a baseball bat and breaking his arm in three places. This was totally out of character, but I can't allow him to take over. If I do, my spirit will be weakened. I may not fight to survive because there is someone there to take care of me.' Given such disastrous consequences, it is hardly surprising if the word 'autonomy' has acquired something of a 'bad press among feminists' (Hampson 1996: 1). Certainly, it merits some clarification: 'to be 'autonomous' is to let one's own law rule one. The word etymologically does not mean independence. It need not imply conceiving of oneself as an isolated atom in competition with others. Indeed, that it has come to hold such connotations may tell us much about the male psyche within patriarchy; as though the only way to be oneself, to take responsibility for oneself, were to set oneself up over against others. No, to be autonomous is to overcome heteronomy. Heteronomy, the law of another ruling one, is the situation of the child' (Hampson 1996: 1).

Although ostensibly expressing the feminist ideal—'I can't allow him to take over', Debbie, like Julia, seems to dangerously imitate the threatened male psyche. Given that the entire history of the development of the Western mind is based on subordinating feminine principles, this ought not to surprise. For a woman caught in the sway of the heroic archetype, there can be an intolerable, confusing, even destructive tension between her conscious analysis of her needs and situation and the promptings of her unconscious mind. In such situations of inner conflict, however, a symbol will sometimes emerge whose function is to reconcile any opposites and to restore psychic order, balance and security (Jacobi 1967: 57–8). Coming to our aid in this manner, the unconscious challenges the rational, conscious mind to understand its symbolic meaning. Debbie, for example, spoke movingly of an 'inner flame'. While recognizing that symbols resist any easy translation, she naturally identified her 'flame' as a source of spiritual support, comfort and daily guidance. 'It's hard to put into words, but it's as though there is a fire burning inside me. It keeps me going. If it's a good day I'll do more, if it's a bad day, I'll do less. The fire inside me, the spirit, allows me to know the difference and to cope. There have been times when my spirit has been really low, like when I came into the hospice. I didn't want to come but I knew I had to. I could feel the flame was going out, that my spirit was weaker. I couldn't walk. I couldn't get out of bed. I couldn't eat. I was just drinking water. Only the spiritual side, my flame, kept me going. I remember the flame was flickering and if it goes out, I don't know if I'll be able to restart.'

A flickering flame can symbolize the raging forest fire as much as the warm glow of hearth and home and Debbie's behaviour certainly fluctuated between extremes of violence and tenderness. Despite resolving to pace herself and conserve her energy, she too required emergency respite care. Perhaps, like Julia, if Debbie had been less committed to the heroic ideal, more accepting of her vulnerabilities and her need for support, she might have fared better. Interestingly, her own solution to her exhaustion is anticipated almost entirely by the earlier feminist analysis of autonomy: 'Only when I came to St Christopher's I felt safe, I felt safe. I had my own room and I thought, "Yeah, this is a nice environment to be in." Staff actually listened to what I would like and did it. It's more of a partnership.'

Another view

When considered as an archetypal symbol, Debbie's 'inner flame' points to the philosophical and theological hinterland of modern psychology. Although adopted by a relatively recent discipline, 'archetype' is far from a modern term.

Even in St Augustine's time it roughly meant the same as Plato's 'idea', the dualistic notion that all phenomena are pre-existed by their perfect concept. Despite the recent trends towards holism in both depth psychology and modern physics, Debbie clearly distinguishes her 'inner' flame from her 'outer' body. The 'outer' form depends upon her 'inner' fire for its well-being, demonstrating how Plato's division clearly still governs popular understandings of body and spirit.

Symbolic meaning, however, confounds transparent categories. It refuses to be encapsulated in ways that ignore subtleties of being and emotion. Soskice (in Hampson 1996: 17) draws a helpful analogy by outlining the difficulties involved in explaining why one might feel in love. Generally speaking, it is not hard to furnish reasons for falling out of love—which is not to say there may be no reasons for loving another. 'Reasons' alone, however, do not keep one in love and neither do they explain why being in love colours one's entire experience. Similarly, symbols both vivify and evade attempts to completely explain their meaning. One has only to recall Moses before the burning bush, the Pentecostal flames, the Hindu practice of Puja, the lighting of the Hebrew Menorah or the baptismal candle, to understand that in all religions the flame is regarded as far more than simply an archetypal product of the psyche. It points to a relationship between finite and infinite. It acts as a mediator for human encounters with the transcendent. Whether signifying love, rage or purification, fire indicates the inherent holiness of life, whilst its destructive capacity provides man with a relativising sense of his place before the ultimate.

Contemporary psychology may sweep aside this ultimate signification, but its own interpretations are frequently no more verifiable than the fourteenth-century writings of Meister Eckhart on the 'divine spark within' (Smith 1987: 108) or for that matter, Debbie's own opinions: 'I have a book with affirmations for everyday that I find very uplifting spiritually. It builds up my self-esteem, my confidence, my flame. Spiritually, it is giving me the motivation to go on. I read it more than I read my Bible now. I've never been one for churches, although I've sort of been searching for a church, but my church is inside and it's about being able to be at peace.'

It is not unreasonable to consider whether Debbie's 'little flame' mediates a spiritual dimension of her experience that extends beyond but also incorporates its psychological interpretation. Neither is it necessary to be even nominally religious to understand that a spiritual interpretation can only address aspects of human experience: motivation, self-esteem, feeling uplifted. It is hard to know what else it can address, for although it attempts to reach the furthest horizon, this always remains ungraspable. In the words of the Buddhist monk Thich Nhat Hanh, 'You cannot describe God. That is why a good theologian is a theologian who almost says nothing of God' (Hanh 1991: 20). Indeed, the only possible verification for the spiritual is one of personal recognition and this only becomes evident to others at a remove, that is, by its consequences or effects in the life of the recognizing individual. For Debbie, the hallmark of authenticity was 'being at peace'. Although she sought and, to some degree, found strength and contentment in her daily reading, Debbie's withdrawal from her marriage and occasional bouts of aggression betray the fragility of these feelings and the mixed potential of her flame. It is a sad irony that over-identification with the hero, with its accompanying and exclusive self-reliance, can be shattering in its consequences, ironic because the heroic narrative may be read as a yearning for wholeness that exceeds processes of psychological maturation. In short, it may be interpreted as an expression of spiritual longing and desire.

Recalling patient's experiences of liminality with their implications of 'somewhere' other than 'here', their increasing feelings of helplessness and the fracturing of the conventional temporal carapace, perhaps a yearning for ultimate security is less than surprising. The Jewish thinker Levinas, finds it hard to understand how, as a finite creature, man's deepest insights can result in anything other than this kind of longing and he writes 'I think that the relation to the Infinite is not a knowledge but a Desire and need, by the fact that Desire cannot be satisfied; that Desire somehow satisfies itself on its own hungers and is augmented by its satisfaction ... It is a paradoxical structure, without doubt, but one which is no more so than this presence of the infinite in a finite act' (Nemo 1985: 92).

Unless a theological perspective accompanies insights afforded by other interpretations of symbols and archetypes, there is a real danger that their full significance will be missed and that the depths of a patient's reality will not be recognized. The possibility that Julia's punishingly positive attitude might veil a deep sense of spiritual dislocation could remain unconsidered. Spiritual hunger as a potential source of domestic violence will fail to register and the notion of mystical presence, the interpenetration of finite and infinite symbolized by fire, is easily passed over. Another consequence of neglecting this ultimate perspective may be that patients feel childish or foolish when they articulate certain intimations or insights or describe certain incidents. With a desire to listen deeply, therefore, we turn to the mediating influence of the archetypal mother.

Archetypal mother

Introduction

Although the heroic life is essentially masculine, patients' attitudes to impending death often include expressions of care and concern for others. A courageous desire to prepare friends, children and other relatives for the inevitable, in the hope of lessening its impact, is not unusual. Careful listening, however, suggests this attitude has less to do with any 'feminizing' of the heroic ideal than with the mediating influence of another archetype: that of the mother. The archetypal mother nurtures and protects, but she is no shining hero, perfection in petticoats. She can be jealous and spiteful. Hera may be the goddess of the home, the guardian of marriage and childbirth and the patron of the family hearth but her hatred was implacable, her jealousies monstrous—all sentiments echoed in Tracey's gentler resentments: 'I don't mind if my husband does remarry, but I don't want her in my house, looking after my kids. Touching my kids. Seeing to my kids. That feels all wrong. I shall always be there looking after them. I ain't never leaving my kids.'

Unlike the hero, who is often portrayed as forever youthful, a *puer aeternus*, the archetypal mother is redolent with ancient wisdom. Aligned with the rhythms of nature she is 'one who knows'. She is the wise old woman of many ancient stories (Estes 1992). Fecundity, nurturance and death are her indivisible aspects and, despite her implications of mortality, the maternal image remains a powerful expression of ultimate reassurance, a comforting guarantor of everything being 'alright'.

Protect and prepare

Perhaps unsurprisingly, younger women especially seemed to derive meaning and purpose from identifying with the archetypal mother. They often described their protection and preparation of others, particularly their children, in quasi-sacrificial terms. Tracey's remarks are not untypical: 'Men keep their identity because they go out to work, but mums are mums all the time. Cancer is such a nasty disease, but you think "better me than one of the kids". Every mother would jump in front of a lorry to save her kid—even if there wasn't a chance. When you take on cancer, it's like you've stepped in front of your kids. It got me, so it can't get them. That's how I feel. Better me than them.'

The careful preparation of friends and family requires delicate and discerning processes, a tricky balancing of current peace of mind against potential future pain. As Camilla put it, 'I try to prepare them, not to scare them. As I deteriorate they'll gradually come to realize.' For many women, gently helping others to accept the inevitability of their dying was a way of preventing future problems and, paradoxically, expressed their commitment to life—even a life in which they could not share: 'Obviously, I want to be here for as long as possible, but I want my son to grow and move on, whether I'm here or not' (Debbie). There is nothing saccharine in the attitude of these women. Their balancing of interests was frequently described as an exhausting responsibility: 'You look at people around you and see them suffering. You think "It's not fair, I can't go yet, I'm going to leave them in too much of a state"' (Tracey). Indeed, the preponderance of orphans in fairy tales suggests that before children can realize their maturity and independence, the idealized ever-sweet mother must die. Nature provides examples of 'tough love' in abundance. She may protect her young ferociously, but the archetypal mother has an unflinching grasp of life's cruelties and the harshness of its lessons. If her offspring are to survive, she knows they must perceive life and death, not simply as opposing realities, but as two aspects of a single thought. Mary describes some of the difficulties involved in realizing this aspiration with her two primary-school-age children, her final sentence conveying urgency and determination: 'It's been hard. I used to say, "Don't worry, I'm not going to die." But then there came a point when I knew I was going to die. We've been very honest and straightforward. They've had to learn that life isn't easy for everyone. Life isn't fair for everyone and they're very unfortunate that it's their mum that's going to die. They've had to come to terms with it. These are deep lessons, but they've no choice. There's no point me saying, "Oh, don't worry, Mummy's going to come home". There is no point in shielding them against something that is going to happen. They have to know, and they have to understand.'

Recalling the prismatic symbol in Fig. 6.1, Mary's argument could be located at the point where the archetypal mother and stranger and metaphors of 'letting go' intersect, for Mary heralds the importance of recognizing what is 'other', even in those with whom we are most familiar. Moreover, as Debbie also illustrates, this is an intersection where Winnicott's (1965a,b) work on the 'good enough' mother provides valuable illumination, closely followed by the contributions of object relations theorists on personality development (Fairbairn 1954; Guntrip 1971): 'Before I took ill, my son was very independent; roller skating, cycling, swimming and so forth. But as soon as I took ill, I was clinging on. He was just as house bound as I was. But now, every time I go to smother him, it's as if my spirit says, "No! Let him go. See what he can do and then see those areas where you can actually help." Instead of doing it for him and not allowing him to do it for himself.'

Believing in preparation as future protection, many women daily performed a delicate balancing act of 'holding' or shielding their children against the future and preparing them for bereavement, between trying to maintain the 'ordinariness' of their lives whilst simultaneously setting up long-term support networks. It is not hard to see why heroic identification is often cited to account for their superhuman efforts. There are, however, other factors pointing to the mediating influence of the archetypal mother.

Rhythms of nature

Unlike their male counterparts, many women referred to the rhythms of nature, the 'life-force', or their own experiences of biological transition. Chuckling as she spoke, Grace recalled her early marriage and her husband's ignorance, 'I'm 80 now, but years ago people knew nothing [i.e. about sexual matters]. We may have married young, but we soon got the hang of it, though I'll never forget the first time my husband saw me have a monthly. I was still asleep. He thought I was bleeding to death and ran straight to get my mother.' Judith, for example, drew a comforting parallel between her earlier fears of childbirth and her current dread of dying, 'It's like when I was expecting the children. There's nothing you can do once you've got so far. You think "I just don't want to go through this". But you know you've got to, so you do. And at the end of it, it's finished, and you do sort of forget about it, I suppose. But you end up with a lovely baby. My biggest fear is still that it's going to be painful— although the doctor has said it shouldn't be.'

Virginity, menstruation, pregnancy, these are the natural limen or thresh- olds of a woman's life with a new beginning underwriting each ending. That a young, terminally ill mother should find the inherently liminal figure of the mermaid significant is unremarkable (Vaughan 1996). Creature of the fron- tier, belonging neither entirely on land nor in the ocean, the mermaid promis- es communication between apparently separate realms. Liminality is her metier and, echoing many of the mothers in this study, Vaughan (once an active medical general practitioner) writes 'I am having a wonderful time fixing treasures for my children, [who] are developing ideas about levels of communication beyond death, which are very exciting to nurture. My spiritual journey is rich and varied and I think that a mother's watching brief passes beyond death' (Vaughan 1996: 565).

Life and death are the two faces of the archetypal mother. In the light of her 'watching brief', frontiers are less absolute. Children were often told that, although their mother would die, her love would never leave them. Much energy was expended in compiling scrapbooks, making videos, in staking some claim in their future. Tracey, for instance, whose family history was not always easy, assumed the status of a guardian angel—again, not saccharine, but faithful to the archetype, promising vengeance should any harm befall her children: 'I will never rest. As soon as they put me in that hole, I'll be out checking and watching over the kids. They say, "Don't you want to go to heaven?" and I say, "No. I'll be too busy down here, even after I'm dead." My poor husband, he thinks, "She ain't ever gonna leave me alone!" I say, "Don't worry, just don't upset my kids." Kids will always need protecting.' Mary also contemplated the 'level' at which she should influence her children's future: 'I've been trying to think of something to leave them, a motto or saying, but end up torn between, "Don't forget your shoes are in the bottom drawer" and "Please remember that Daddy loves you, despite the fact he shouts at you." I don't know at what level one should reflect on life and leave thoughts behind, or even if it's unfair; people do have to manage without me. I was making a video of me at every stage. Every time I switched the thing on I said, "I'm not really sure why I'm doing this", but it was to leave to my children.' Debbie hoped to visit her son in his dreams, sustaining him much as she felt supported by her late father. 'My son will ask, "Did you dream about Grand-Dad, because you woke happier today? Next time, send him my love." We are quite open about it and I think that helps.'

The archetypal mother does not deny death, but clearly she resists its exclusively medical definition. Her favouring of cyclical movement, seasons, transition and fecundity over linear representation and finality intimates horizons beyond the conventional medical frontier. As Tracey here illustrates, this reinforces metaphor as an agent in any linguistics of spirit: 'I said to the kids I won't be able to see you as I see you now, but I will be with you, for as long as you keep going. And when you have kids, they'll be a part of me. My life never ends. I see a light so I see where I'm going. When I die I'll see a light so I know where I'm going.'

The desire to nurture and comfort, however, was not exclusively reserved for offspring. Judith worried more for her husband than for her children, whom she regarded as 'old enough to make their own way. They're not being left orphaned, not like little ones. It's my husband I feel sorry for because he is going to be alone.' Irene hoped both to reconcile her sister with the earlier loss of a daughter and to prevent a similarly pained bereavement in her own husband after her own death: 'It's done my sister good to talk, even though she had counselling. But my husband, no, he won't need counselling, because he's been prepared in advance.' Camilla shielded her 'macho' but vulnerable ex-boyfriend with her dry humour, sometimes using flippancy to 'get over certain points'. Preparing and waiting for 'right times', the archetypal mother realizes the dangers of premature parturition or forced confrontation. Camilla thus patiently accepted that her ex was a 'very private person who doesn't show much', but still hoped he would 'get better, not so macho, so uptight as time goes along. Men don't cry in his book, which is a load of baloney. But that's the way he is, and he is, slowly, getting better.'

Insofar as the desires of Camilla, Judith, Tracey and many women focus on defusing the chaotic emotions of others, on sustaining, protecting or preparing loved ones, they imply some awareness of life possessing an ultimately 'proper' design and order characterized by peace and well-being. This awareness transcends the messily near at hand and may be regarded as another 'rumour of angels' (Berger 1969). Certainly, for many of the women, this propensity to order required a view wider than their immediate circumstances. Fantasies or dreams of the future were not uncommon. Tracey often imagined her children 'grown up and with their own lives. But I'm not in those dreams. I'm not there. It's like watching a film, only I'm not in it. When I wake up I feel good because I know they're gonna be alright.' Mary even wondered whether her dying was something 'meant to be', perhaps influencing one of her children to eventually become 'something like a research scientist.' Convinced that her early death was for some reason, part of an ordered process, 'even if I can't see it', she found even the possibility of a wider picture a comforting source of meaning and purpose. Unfortunately, however, such a perspective is no guarantee of happiness or an easeful path to death.

Costs

Just as heroic identification sometimes enables ordinary people to perform extraordinary feats, many of the women whose reality was mediated by maternal metaphor displayed tremendous endurance and grit: 'Whenever my spirit gets really low, I think of my son. I want to live so much to see him grow and become independent' (Debbie). The costs involved in being a 'good enough' mother, coupled with the searing knowledge of inevitable separation, are inestimable: 'even though he's grown, I just want to take him to me breast and hold him there forever' [making a stroking movement with one hand over her breast] (Josie). Capability can be extended beyond the point of endurance.

Sadness and exhaustion can overwhelm. As Tracey explained, 'the hardest part is keeping everyone else OK. If you become ill, then everybody falls like a deck of cards; they don't act normal, they don't talk normal. I'm just holding up, but [beginning to cry] I just wanna lay down.' Gasping for breath, Mary also explained, 'My eldest one, she's nine and more emotional. At bedtime she starts getting sad. You get a big sad face and the sincere cuddles and you think "I don't need this now."'

Although each of these women wanted their experiences to help others, personal need may also have been a motivating factor to participate in this research. Debbie, for example, said she, 'longed for this sort of conversation'. Sighing deeply, but still concerned to protect her family from her own distress, Tracey acknowledged her need 'for an outlet to give me a break, to get me out of here. The only people I talk with are St Christopher's. I can cry if I want to, but I won't have my husband in the house then, or my kids. You need someone from outside.'

Although the desire to protect family members was strong, attitudes towards husbands and partners were sometimes ambivalent, tinged with frustration or disappointment. Tracey's guarding brief has been noted. Debbie felt harassed and burdened by her husband's distress. Although Mary spoke of making a video to leave her children, in the context of her obvious irritation with her husband's poor domestic abilities, his unemployment and short temper, her description reads as a more diffuse vote of 'no confidence': 'Provided my husband isn't entirely stupid, he may be able to put the original onto the official tape … but there's trouble with his ability … he may lose the whole thing … he doesn't know. He's not very good at handling …' [voice fading to silence].

Of course, emotionally and physically exhausted carers will sometimes fail but perhaps a woman's identification with the archetypal mother actually prevents her partner from exercising his full supportive capacity. The potency of this archetype is such that she virtually eclipses the masculine—much as Debbie refused to allow her husband to attend her hospital appointments. Alternatively, it may be that there is greater need for this archetype to mediate the experiences of an inadequately supported woman. The strength, meaning and purpose with which events are framed may be more vital. Josselson (1996a: 35) recalls earlier discussions of control and the human need for security: 'Falling is one of the most terrifying of sensations … an experience of utter loss of control … of complete helplessness and powerlessness … The holding experience is a complicated one to understand because it is neither cognitively realistic nor emotionally intelligible. The sense of holding exists between fantasy and reality: we feel held even though we know that we are not.

We rely on people even though we know that they cannot promise us safety. It is the juxtaposition of our knowing and not knowing that gives our need to be held its distinctive cast.'

To distinguish 'fantasy' from 'reality' in this way, however, is naïve; there is no unmediated access to reality. Understanding is not simply a matter of grasping established 'facts'. It involves knowing what something means, possessing a sympathetic awareness. Expressed in these terms, even infants may understand. The 'holding experience' is thus intelligible, if not always explicable. D. H. Lawrence's (1993: 88) wonderful evocation of the secure child shows how meaning provides protection without necessarily offering explanation: 'She looked from one to the other, and she saw them as established to her safety and she was free ... Her father and her mother now met to the span of the heavens, and she, the child, was free to play in the space beneath, between.' To 'understand' whilst 'not knowing' is an unabashedly Augustinian paradox and paradox is part of the vocabulary of spirit. The way in which the archetypal mother mediates Tracey and her children's response to her illness highlights aspects of their experience that, to evoke an older connotation, 'stand under' a theological interpretation, at least as comfortably as under any other.

The 'absent presence'

During one respite admission, Tracey described how her children were coping with her absence: 'They've made this model of me, this statue cardboard thing of me that says I'm there, even when I'm not there. It was their idea, not mine. So, when Mum's not there, this thing takes over. It's a great big thing. It's got my hair, my clothes and things like that. It stands about 6 feet tall in the corridor. No one touches it, no matter what. If I'm out, it's always there to remind us: this is me. And when I go away, I think they look at it a lot more.' Proud of her children's creative endeavour, Tracey invited me to take some photographs (Fig. 11.1).

The statue, towering majestic in a corner of her hall, was surrounded by the usual paraphernalia of family life: a football, children's shoes, carrier bags—as well as the less familiar nebulizer. Carefully situated opposite the front door and at the foot of the stairs, the children had ensured its surveillance of every movement in the small flat.

This interesting scenario is illuminated by a variety of psychological theory related to child development. Spontaneous play often fosters personal growth, nurtures group relationships and diffuses the threatening (Klein 1988: 16). Always lively, it is easy to imagine the children feeling so entranced, so totally absorbed in play that they entered a safe 'potential space' or area of experiencing that mediates between inner and outer realities (Winnicott 1971).

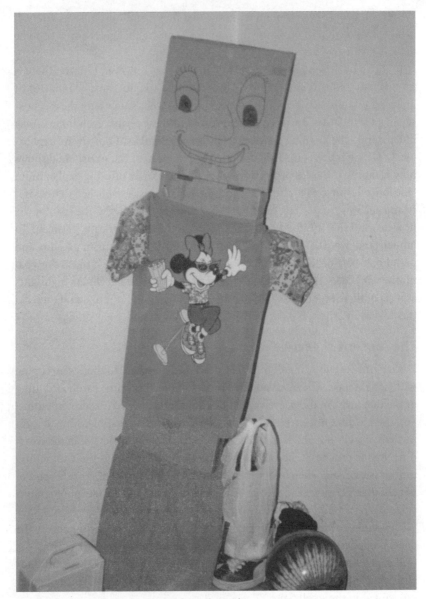

Figure 11.1 Tracey's statue. (See Colour Plate 7.)

Obliquely acknowledging their sad situation together in this space was perhaps comforting. The products or tools of play sometimes act as 'transitional objects' forming a link between one person and another. Gradually, they enable younger children to learn to separate from their mother. Clearly representing Tracey's love and security in her absence, the statue may also be considered in these terms and the creative activity whereby it was produced as 'a process [which] enables us to absorb experience with our whole being, to give it a form and shape, thereby enhancing our capacity to live. By gaining conscious control of unconscious imagery we bring into order our own chaotic psyches. It is a process of self -healing. In art you are able to give expression to that which lies deep inside you, and having given expression to it, you receive back a vision which is a map by which you can set your other goals' (Roose-Evans 1994: 153).

Tracey's use of the third person when speaking of the statue ('it's for when Mum's not home') creates the sense of something 'larger than life', hinting at its archetypal significance. Inevitably, this prompts a Jungian interpretation, tantalizing in its proximity to the overtly theological: 'For centuries humans have felt that dolls emanate both a holiness and a *mana*—an awesome and compelling prescience which acts upon persons changing them spiritually … Dolls are believed to be infused with life by their makers. They are used in rites, ritual, voodoo, love spells, and mischief. The doll is the symbolic *homunculi*, little life. It is the symbol of what lies buried in humans that is numinous. It is a small and glowing facsimile of the original Self. Superficially, it is just a doll, but in the doll is the voice of the One Who Knows' (Estes 1992: 88). From Estes's Jungian perspective, however, this voice is unequivocally human. Other than in terms of collective consciousness, there are no grounds from which she argues for the transcendent. Any theological contemplation of that of 'me' which may also be 'other' is fruitless because 'whether the psychic structure and its elements, the archetypes, ever "originated" at all is a metaphysical question, and, therefore, unanswerable' (Jung 1996: 101). This dogmatic severance, however, is unsatisfactory and two questions immediately arise: 'Answerable according to whose criteria?' and 'What is the function of any answer?' Surely 'answers' function to deepen our understanding of what is happening in a given situation and understanding does not owe its allegiance to any one particular way of knowing. Augmented, understanding enables us to relate to one another more humanely. We 'read' encounters with greater insight and deeper satisfaction. We have a clearer sense of what is going on and, more importantly, a better idea of who we are. The horizons of developmental psychology, psychotherapeutic theory, sociology or anthropology entice and inform but they are not the widest. The children's 'goddess of the home' invites a more radical interpretation. The religious and artistic connotations of Tracey's own terminology ('statue'), coupled with the taboo against any tampering, distinguish the cardboard, crayoning, plastic bottles and old clothes from the normal detritus of childhood activity. At some level, this suggests these trivia have been discerned as a disclosure point for some extra-mundane dimension of reality. The answer to Jung's metaphysical question lies not in the scientific method, but in an understanding of what it means to take part in ritual, to live sacramentally.

Creative activity: sacramental awareness

Although sacraments and the sacramental have come to be regarded as synonymous with religious rite, acting as visible signs and channels for supernatural grace, it is possible to appeal to all aspects of human experience in sacramental terms. It is from this argument that we approach Tracey's statue: that sacrament touches everything that is 'distinctly human'; that the sacramental makes individuals and society the more 'truly human' insofar as it fosters self-reflection and facilitates a movement towards others in love (Cooke 1983: 2). In short, the children's creative enterprise manifests that sacraments are not 'magical' events but 'moments of reflection, shared with one another in celebration, that bring together and deepen all our reflections about life' (Cooke 1983: 12).

To be concerned with the sacramental, therefore, is to be concerned with interpreting human experience at its deepest level, a level which addresses the whole person not simply the intellect. From the Latin *ex per*, experience means to learn by trying out and extended, *per* becomes *periculum*, meaning trial, danger, peril. Similarly, the Greek *peira* (origin of fare and ferry) expresses notions of movement and risk. It is possible to interpret the making of the statue in these dynamic terms. Painful emotions may have been diffused, difficult realizations expressed safely in the 'space' created by the children's creative activity, but this was not without danger. Arguments, emotional trauma and tears are rarely distant when children play—perhaps never more so than when creating a symbol of their dying mother. The siblings, however, passed beyond these dangers until their statue became a comforting and protective presence. For a child, there are perhaps few periods more liminal than the final stages of their mother's life and whether spontaneous (as in this case) or formal, the collective ritual has long provided a means of safely approaching such frontiers.

Culturally determined, formal rituals mark significant transitions—weddings, births, deaths—and embody a particular vision of life. The creation of the statue may be considered as a spontaneous engagement in informal ritual. Although, in both instances, ordinary things—clothes or food, cardboard or plastic bottles—mediate an extraordinary meaning, some words of caution should be registered. The idea of the ordinary acting as a window upon the transcendent can foster dualistic concepts such as the notion of a supernatural realm lying 'behind' or 'beyond' immediate appearances. Certainly, the ordinary may lead to a vision of the extraordinary, but there are not two worlds where the latter is 'hidden' behind the former. Human experience is better understood as a series of symbol systems. The symbol does not permit any division of the ultimate or spiritual from the mundane. This is because the symbol embodies the reality it mediates. Although no symbol ever totally embodies the transcendent, understanding a symbol is not a matter of reading meaning 'in', but of reading 'out' what is already there. Even so, the deepest meaning of a symbol or symbolic action is rarely immediately recognized. Rather, understanding gradually crystallizes and it resists attempts to render it explicit. Thus, music, poetry or art have to be understood on their own terms. Similarly, effective ritual sustains and nourishes at subconscious and emotional levels as much as at the cognitive, continuing to do so long after its participants have dispersed. Consider the Last Supper where 'Jesus ... got up from table, removed his outer garment and taking a towel, wrapped it around his waist; he then poured water into a basin and began to wash the disciples feet and to wipe them with the towel he was wearing. He came to Simon Peter who said to him, "Lord, are you going to wash my feet?" Jesus answered, "At the moment, you do not know what I am doing, but later you will understand"' (*John* Chapter 13, Verses 6–7). For Tracey's children, similar processes of 'learning from' making their statue are involved, rather than 'learning about' anything. With this kind of knowledge 'we learn by doing in the same way [as] we make a path by walking. It is in the nature of ritual to lead one across the threshold of liminality into an experience of gnosis of insight' (Roose-Evans 1994: 81).

Any future reflections the children might make upon the statue would certainly be of interest. Although grounded in their distressing situation, the duration of its symbolic potency is unpredictable. As Tracey understood, 'They'll just know when it's time to put it away.' All that can be said with any certainty is that 'if ritual remains alive it is because the symbolisms in it are truly effective' (Cooke 1983: 40) ... 'They must be truly living symbols. They must genuinely relate to the realities of our human experience; they must spring from and remain in contact with that experience' (Cooke 1983: 49). Lest such arguments appear to exaggerate the significance of a simple act of play, it is helpful to recall other informal but less remarkable rituals. Each helped to make a patient's situation more tolerable, lending credence to the notion of a 'surplus of meaning' residing in even the simplest action: Carol gazing each evening at her 'guiding beacon' the Crystal Palace aerial; Arthur standing stiffly to attention, saluting each man who left his bay for the mortuary; even Debbie's decision to cut her hair has a deeper resonance, symbolizing her desire to 'take control'.

Thus far, depth psychology and theological interpretation are in accordance. The critical point of divergence again centres on the source of symbolic potency. Unlike the psychologist, whose interest is purely anthropological, the theologian also considers the world in terms of its ultimate grounding. Theologically speaking, 'all ritual, should give expression to the deepest yearning within us, urging us towards something that always remains beyond us' (Roose-Evans 1994: 49). From this perspective, although in the making of their statue, personal and interpersonal dimensions embrace, Tracey's children also find themselves standing in some personal relation to an apparently limitless capacity of knowing and loving. The audacity of this claim is sustained only by the degree to which they manifest the beneficial consequences of their play and the extent to which they demonstrate a sense of feeling strangely understood. This is where something makes sense not to us, but in us, at a level lying deeper than the furthest reaches of our creative capacity. When Tracey was asked what she thought her children might do with the statue should she suddenly die, she responded 'At the moment, its just part of the furniture. I don't know what they're going to do with it when I die. I don't want them to hold on to the cardboard figure. I want them to have the memories inside their head, because anything can happen. If they had a ring of mine, they could lose it. I don't want them to be so upset they're thinking, "Oh God, I've lost my Mum's ring", or anything like that. I want whatever memories they've got inside their head. It doesn't have to be anything solid or a picture of me.'

This answer invites a classical Jungian interpretation as a statement about processes of individuation (becoming personally whole) and personal integration. Tracey knows that her children need to internalize the qualities they attribute to the statue to find and stabilize their own inner source of security. As Jung explains, 'an archetype is in no sense just an annoying prejudice; it becomes so only when it is in the wrong place. Our task is not to deny the archetype, but to dissolve the projections, in order to restore their contents to the individual who has involuntary lost them by projecting them outside himself' (Jung 1996: 84). For object relation theorists, the children will instinctively know when to put the statue aside, recognizing that such play is no longer necessary to 'carry' them to a safer space. As an object of transference, the statue becomes redundant.

Notwithstanding the value of these interpretations, however, there is much in Tracey's comments about the statue, personal mortality and childhood bereavement that merits further consideration. Certainly, hers is an injunction against idolatry, or any estimation of the false, in favour of the authentic. She knows that the truths whereby her children will most happily live must come from within. Other sources are precarious. As she said, 'anything can happen'. Human fidelity, symbolized by the easily misplaced ring, is subject to the vicissitudes of life. Instinctively, therefore, she knows that the greatest danger for her children lies in confusing the ultimate source of security with the conditional. Expressed theologically, 'It is the danger of every embodiment of the unconditioned element, religious and secular, that it elevates something conditioned, a symbol, an institution, a movement, as such, to Ultimacy' (Tillich 1964*b*: 29).

Tracey both realizes and demonstrates this in her appeal to truth and constancy. Desiring her children's lives to embody these values is but a contemporary rendition of the parable of the two houses: one built on sand, the other rock (*Luke* Chapter7, Verses 47–8). The shared symbolic value of the children's play and the parable, however, does not only yield to a psychological 'translation'. The wholeness and perfection of the qualities that Tracey hopes for exceeds human capability. This she obliquely acknowledges with her comment on the statue: 'it's me and it's not me.' Given her ambitions for her children, the 'not me' thus invokes a sense of largesse, as well as difference. The height of these aspirations expresses a confidence in something even the most perfect mother may not embody. As such, they are a form of blessing whose understanding exceeds the parameters of any non-theological interpretation and whose realization through the children's play will always be something of a mystery. The healing of separation, whether inter- or intra-personal, is the ultimate function of ritual: '"Never!" said Peter, "You shall never wash my feet". Jesus replied, "If I do not wash you, you can have nothing in common with me"' (*John* Chapter 4, Verse 8).

To engage with any ritual, secular or religious, at this depth of fulfilment is a form of prayer. One is open to and flooded by a positive potential for transformation. The deepest meaning of the children's play, their utter absorption in their activity; their transportation to a 'safe space' and its beneficial consequences, emerges from understanding their game as a non-religious expression of prayer. They touch a horizon which is only partially embodied by the psyche, and it heals. Much as we continuously, often unconsciously, live and reveal our physical or emotional dimensions, the same is true of our spiritual. It may remain largely tacit, but a combination of human and ultimate concern exists, not only in the children's creativity, but also in Tracey's interpretation of their play. Perhaps mother and children would be surprised to hear what psychologists, sociologists or theologians make of their statue, but there can be no denial of the reverence and affection it inspired, the love and devotion it symbolized. The following story—not entirely dissimilar from that recounted here—illustrates that the spiritually significant may be more comprehensively mediated by values than by 'facts', by the illogical than the rational. By so doing, it also furnishes an appropriate conclusion to these discussions: 'A woman of great devotion asked her son, who frequently went to India on business, to bring her a sacred object from the land of Buddha—India. The son forgot about it until he got close to home. He took the tooth from the corpse of a dog, wrapped it up in brocade and silk, and handed it to his mother saying, "Mother I brought a tooth of the Buddha to be the object of your homage." For the rest of her life the mother worshipped the tooth with total belief and devotion as if it were a true tooth of the Buddha. From the tooth miraculous signs appeared, and at the time of her death rainbow lights arched over her body as a sign of high spiritual attainment' (Paltrul Rinpoche in Thundup 1996: 94).

Chapter 12

Archetypal stranger

Inherent tensions

As with mother and hero, the stranger emerges as an archetypal product of the psyche and as a linguistic phenomenon involving archetypal metaphors. Challenging the post-Descartian mind, the metaphor and psychic construct each invoke ambiguity, fluidity and the strain of the relational. *Extraneous*, the Latin origin of 'stran', suggests the foreigner, the outsider, the potentially threatening. 'Ger', *gwr* in Hebrew, points to traditions of protection and receptivity, 'Thou shalt not hate an Egyptian for thou wast a stranger in his land' (*Deuteronomy* Chapter 23, Verse 8), where hospitality demonstrates fidelity to the covenant, a recognition of ultimate concern (*Wisdom* Chapter 11, Verses 24–7) and, as Abraham's reception of unknown travellers demonstrates (*Genesis* Chapter 18, Verses 1–15), a realization that although the stranger may threaten, he can also bear gifts. The Greek *xenodochius* (from *xenodokheion*)— a hostel or reception centre for strangers—enlarges meaning yet further. *Xenos* (stranger) signifies pilgrimage, quest and processes of becoming.

Perhaps this challenge of the relational accounts for the scant attention paid in palliative literature to the stranger. Hero and mother are more easily conceptualized, whereas the dialectics invoked by the figure of the stranger resist categorization. Even a cursory inspection of patient narrative and experience, however, renders this oversight unjustifiable. The phenomena of estrangement overshadow, and are influenced by, nearly every other facet of our prism— especially those concerning marginality, liminality and time. Falling in line with a generalized contemporary preoccupation with 'otherness', whether expressed sociologically through research into the experiences of minority groups or emerging in existential literature such as Camus's (1981), *L'Etranger* (the outsider), each etymological nuance can be argued from patient experience. Contemporary theory, however, handles estrangement obliquely, if at all. Jungian psychology approaches it in terms of the shadow (Jung 1996: 20), sociology, in terms of generality and specificity of characteristics (Wolff 1950) and theology, via discussions of essential nature (Tillich 1964*b*) or man's relationship with a transcendent Other (Llewelyn 1995; Levinas in Nemo 1985), merging with considerations of alterity and the foreign in philosophy (Waldenfels 1996).

In the face of such diversity, the primary concern here nevertheless remains the range of existential commitment in each of these approaches, the degree to which they are brought to mind by patients' experiences and how successfully they accommodate 'the stranger' as an expression and mediator of the dying person's reality and their spiritual needs. Mindful of this, despite the multiplicity of perspectives, two themes highlighting specific tensions emerge in virtually all disciplines and are clearly identifiable in patient narrative and behaviour: non-recognition of one's own self and non-recognition of oneself by others.

Near but far

Descriptions of personhood tend to rely upon the *via negative*. Terms such as 'individual' or 'integrated', for example, stem from the Latin *in dividere*, meaning indivisible and *in tangere*, not touched. This suggests that recognition should be conceptualized in terms of accessibility rather than of possession. Sociologically, processes of recognition inextricably co-exist with those of estrangement forming a tense and fluid relationship (Simmel 1950: 402). The stranger is simultaneously both far and near. Differing in specific ways from the general norm, he is a distant figure but, because strangers are always recognized as strangers of a particular type, he is also near. Irene both witnessed, and vigorously resisted, such typecasting: 'in my camping group, I'm the second one to have cancer. I've kept it low key because I know that if Pat came camping, everyone watched her every move. I want to be treated normal. There will be people who won't know about it until I've actually died. I told one friend who said "I got a book and read up all about it. I know what all your symptoms are."' Earlier discussions of liminality come to mind, for both the inaccessibility of the stranger's situation and their relational existence are illustrated here. As she explains, for Irene to cross the threshold that distinguished her from others would require her to become, if only momentarily, someone else: 'I'm looking from the inside out, rather than from the outside in. If you had cancer, well, things would be completely different. I'm looking at it from my side, where I've got it, and you haven't. You can't really understand if you haven't got it.' Paradoxically, of course, some degree of inaccessibility is always necessary when considering those who differ from the norm, otherwise the more their situation is explained, the more their 'otherness' risks being silenced or undermined by studies that actually destroy that which they seek to understand.

To recognize is not simply to label or appropriate by naming, for names are not synonymous with lists of characteristics—just as knowledge of another does not equate with a recounting of their deeds. To call by name, however, does imply some degree of recognition, for changes in name can indicate shifts in identity, rather than simply in title. The fairy tale character Rumpelstiltskin illustrates a common cultural association between revealing one's name and becoming vulnerable. Recognition, however, concerns not only the one who is named but carries implications for the namer. A mutuality of giving and receiving may be involved. Assumption of one's 'true' or more complete (as distinct from 'false') status or identity sometimes requires recognition by another, an ability on their part to penetrate or 'see beyond' the seemingly obvious. It is worth considering the experience of Eileen and her husband in the light of de Hennezel's (1997: 181) claim that 'dignity is not given, but seen in another.' After her partial mastectomy Eileen wanted to see her husband's reaction: 'I wouldn't even look at it, but once I got his reaction, I was alright. He was very good about it, very good.'

Perhaps Eileen's husband, as much as Eileen herself, was bound up in a process of becoming. Only after identifying Christ, could Simon become Peter; only after enlightenment was Gautama known as the Buddha. Self-actualization often involves wounding and struggle. Presumably Eileen's mastectomy was a source of distress to her husband. Certainly, his response to the distressingly unfamiliar was a critical moment, a moment as radical in its consequences, perhaps, as Jacob's encounter at the ford of Jabbok where he too received a new name. Finally, personal reflection on the hours of conversation that went towards the making of this book endorses the view that 'the stranger summons us to change, to rethink our own identities, to reorder our cherished priorities' (Nicholls 1995: 14).

The stranger always implies the tensions of relationality, but it is important to remember that 'he' is not necessarily encountered in the guise of another. For Hazel, 'when someone said that a certain path wasn't made for the handicapped, it gave me a shock. I don't think of myself as being handicapped but, of course, I am.' Sick or not, few people have never been surprised by their own reflection or by another's assessment of their character. Complete knowledge either of oneself or another is elusive. We are not exhaustively accessible. With internal and external processes of estrangement and intimacy continually shifting and mutually implicating, there is a sense in which I am not entirely master of myself. Sometimes, 'it is someone else's gaze that brings me into being' (de Hennnezel 1997: 54). From a linguistic perspective, because it is impossible not to communicate (no response is a response), a certain distance or estrangement from sources of personal initiative and choice is again implied. If the external stranger is one who is familiar but different, near but far, it would seem that a similar tension links the 'work of alterity in the heart of selfhood' (Ricoeur 1992: 368).

Whilst recognizing that a sick person may need to evade certain truths to cope, psychological perspectives on estrangement sometimes focus on how personal defences can obstruct processes of self-recognition. Recollecting the havoc brought about by patients' excessive identification with an idealized heroic, however, also demonstrates the significance of the archetypal shadow in processes of self-estrangement, where everything an individual refuses to accept or recognize about themselves, they tend to project on to others. It is difficult to escape the conclusion that something of the stranger exists in each of us. Inexhaustible in its imagery, our personal subconscious defies appropriation whilst the collective unconscious is remarkable for its universal, yet simultaneously alienating qualities. It 'no sooner touches us than we are it, we become unconscious of ourselves' (Jung 1996: 22)—hence those adventurers in fairy tales who, on breaching the castle ramparts or on penetrating the dark wood (both symbolic of entering the unconscious) immediately fall into a deep sleep.

Hazel's interesting compound of the unconventional and the archaic, however, suggests that perhaps sociological and psychological understandings of otherness or estrangement can only take one so far. For Hazel, 'God is a divine and heavenly psychiatrist, someone who knows me completely and from whom no hearts are hid.' Psychology provides many valuable insights into the human need for 'unconditional positive regard' (Rogers 1980) and Hazel certainly expresses a deep human need to be unconditionally known and accepted. Her appeal, however, also has a spiritual dimension for it stems from an experience of finitude when the preferred experience is one of infinite love. This desire is the theological horizon tacitly implied and contained in the moment Eileen's husband responded to her surgery. Hazel articulates the same need to be loved but she makes explicit the ultimate perspective by using religious terminology. For both women risk is involved: human love is fallible— Eileen's husband could have pulled a face, turned away. The Ultimate horizon, as Hazel found, differs from no other in being ever approachable but never attainable; the degree to which it is 'possessed' is determined only by the perspective it provides to a tangible foreground, existentially, in situations such as the one in which Eileen and her husband found themselves.

Theological and psychological interpretations of human experience often overlap but they are not always equivalent. Judith, for instance, who always felt she 'could have done better' illustrates much contemporary theory on the development of self-worth, although her own interpretation of her situation and what it required rely upon notions of revelation and gift before those of personal development: 'God must have a reason for doing this. I keep hoping that one day something will sort of show me.' This is not to say that the contributions of psychology are irrelevant, far from it, but perhaps intimates a more radical tension that may not simply be dismissed.

It is Tillich (1964a) who makes the audacious existential claim, who performs from a theological perspective what Jung, when he points to all religious experience of the numinous as rooted in the impact of the collective unconscious, achieves from the psychological. For Tillich, man is driven to recover his essential humanity, from which he is estranged, but never fully severed. Expressed eternally in God, any sense man has of the ultimate is possible only because he is grounded therein. The presupposition of any search for God, therefore, is an ambiguous possession of and by him. For such knowledge, however, one can only wait. Beyond a certain level, investigating existence does not produce the answer to its problem. As Judith seems to understand, 'God is the answer to the question implied in human finitude. This answer cannot be derived from the analysis of existence ... revelation is 'spoken' to man but not by man himself" (Tillich 1964c 64–5). Our concern is with whether the tensions experienced by terminally ill people extend to these ultimate, yet paradoxically intimate, horizons. In short, with whether it is justifiable to present this analysis of the stranger as a work of theological anthropology, an exploration of finitude, as well as supporting its sociological or psychological implications.

Waiting: source of ultimate tension

Waldenfels (1996: 115) writes 'The place that includes me and excludes the other is appropriated at the same moment. It is occupied as my point of view, my residence, my habits. The unity of these forms ... is one's own body as anchorage in the world.' It is hardly surprising, therefore, if dissolution of the body, whether by illness or by accident, has implications more profound than the merely physical. To be facing death is to occupy a position of acute tension and maintaining any sense of personal security may become impossible. As Hazel found, 'It's like being totally churned upside down. Like the jars in the botany class that you had to shake and then watch everything settle to see what they were made of.'

Many changes in conviction or lifestyle are preceded by a period of estrangement and of becoming, when the significance of all that has been seems to dissolve, yet one has not fully entered a new mode of existence. This situation is often hallmarked by the discomforting sense of something happening 'now' but 'not yet'. There is a suspended sense of anticipation and waiting. Encounters where one experiences estrangement as *extraneous* may magnify this tension and the trauma of such waiting may pierce so deeply that immediate relief seems only to lie in precipitating the apparently inevitable. In Jane's case this meant taking her own life before falling entirely prey to motor neurone disease. Speaking bitterly, she remarked 'I went to an MND meeting. Lots were in wheelchairs, not able to speak. I looked at them and thought "No way am I going to end up like this." I'd already lost the use of one arm. So I took an overdose but they found me and pumped me out, brought me through.' Sooner or later, most hospice patients encounter someone for whom the 'not yet' of dying becomes the 'now' of death. Although a paradoxical mixture of comfort, distress and lower levels of depression have been reported amongst patients who witness another person die (Payne *et al.* 1996), some people clearly regard the experience negatively. Julia found it 'very hard to stay positive when two out of four of you die, to say to yourself "I'm not going down that road, not this time."' Jane's most recent respite admission 'wore me right down. Opposite, were two elderly ladies. You could see they were dying; moaning and groaning. I went right down, worse than when I come in. Every time I opened my eyes, there were these two faces opposite me. When you see them lain there dying and you're not, it sends you deep. I just thought, "I'm not gonna get out of here."'

The depth to which Jane alludes cannot be ignored by any study of human spirituality for it often draws those who enter it towards at least two profound existential questions. These are 'Who am I?' and 'Am I related to anything infinite or not?' Furthermore, ex-nurses Jane and Camilla are valuable reminders that health professionals may be less, not more, able to cope with sickness and mortality. For them, death may be a 'familiar stranger', but repeated encounters do not necessarily diminish its threatening capacity: 'I've seen a lot of people die and that's for sure. I was only 20 and when my friend and I came on duty, someone had always just died. We would have to do the last wash. We totted up how many we did over 4 months. I did 60. Ever since then, I don't like anything to do with death or with dead bodies. It's horrible. There was no counselling or anything like that then, you just had to get on with it' (Camilla).

The inherent tensions of 'now but not yet' echo in metaphors of liminality and letting go. They may be heard both in Arthur's stoic resignation and in Mary and Carol's optimism. Respectively, these attitudes may be framed in terms of coping with danger or personifying the unknown in terms of *xenos,* a pilgrimage or journey and *gwr,* as carrying some benign potential. In a period more naturally associated with decline, taking life's potential for gift to its furthest existential reach passes a point where human and ultimate concerns converge. Although Hazel's language is religious (the vocabulary of the second-order proposition), 'There is still time for God to take me under his wing and for me to know that—whether it will happen or not, I can't tell', her feelings of estrangement, her uncertainty and her need for a comfort and support larger than present circumstances repeatedly occurred. Metaphors of estrangement carry psychological and inter-relational implications but pursued to their extreme, they point in the direction of theological territory and the human need for ultimate reassurance. In terms of first-order propositions, many terminally ill people seem to navigate this terrain using a compass marked with questions of meaning and purpose.

Self as stranger

Ill health and suffering force individuals to face new or unrecognizable aspects of self. Julia presents the case concisely: 'I resent being sick because I don't feel this is me.' The subtle and not so subtle shifts occasioned by terminal illness, however, seem to emphasize the 'non-self', the 'me-that-is-not-me', distorting even the most primordial form of alterity; the customary rapport between one's flesh and one's body. Wasted and scarred, struggling into the bath, for example, an ex-dancer sighed 'I can't believe this is me. I was so strong, so fit, so supple.' Physical deterioration furnishes brutal introductions. Jane's suspicions of serious illness were aroused by an unfamiliar reflection: 'I looked in the mirror and I noticed there was slight wastage in the shoulder. I thought "that's not right, that shoulder's not right."' Camilla was alarmed when her knees felt 'like cotton wool' and Irene as she gradually realized 'I'm shorter. I've lost a couple of inches. Also, I wasn't round shouldered before, but now I have to droop my shoulders to take the strain off my back.' Each woman expresses a sense of personal dislocation, of no longer feeling 'at home' in her own body. Certainly, radical surgery, disability and disfigurement can restrict self-expression, undermine self-confidence and diminish feelings of sexual appeal and vitality (Yaniv 1995). Eileen found 'The mastectomy distresses me, especially when I go to buy clothes. I can't buy things that are sleeveless, because it's all puckered under my arm. You put your arm up and it's horrible, like a rock, really hard, like a rock.'

Carla drew a sad comparison between the faces of her visitors when they entered her side room and that of her husband when they were first married. Clearly neither she, nor they, regarded her as the same woman. Using a vibrant colourful picture (Fig. 12.1), in direct contrast with the neutrality of her side room, she explained how she would once wait, joyfully naked, for her husband to enter their bedroom. Following her mastectomy, however, she too felt

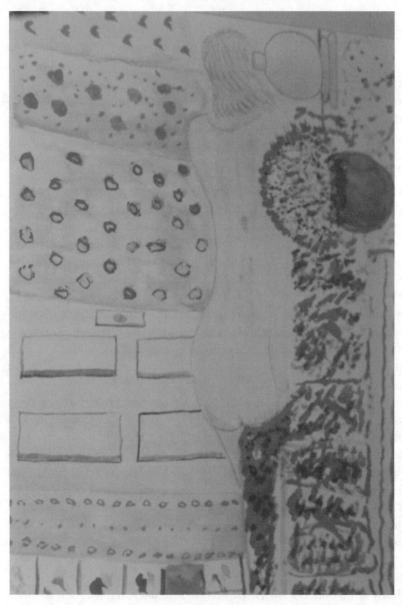

Figure 12.1 Reclining nude. (See Colour Plate 8.)

'unfeminine, I didn't want my husband to look at my body. He assured me that it wasn't a problem between us and he still loved me, whatever. But I still felt that, with only having one breast, I felt bad. I still feel lopsided and not quite feminine, even today.'

Although less documented amongst men, feelings of loss and diminution, are not confined to women. Dependency affronts masculinity and restricts access to gender-biased activities such as sport. For instance, Gregory was 'very, very sporty all my life, and fit with it. I thoroughly enjoyed it. It makes the physical changes so hard to believe. God it's hard. I was pretty proud of my physique really. I had a good physique, strong too. Yes, a bit of male vanity … [voice fading].' Gregory's blindness removed him from an immediately accessible, specifically male, world. To interpret his proclaimed but questionable adjustments as macho posturing is too simple: 'I don't know, call it the human spirit, it comes to terms with that sort of thing.' Ricoeur (1992) suggests a more sensitive route; masculine pride, as much as woman's sexual confidence, actually requires some degree of 'fundamental alterity', some sense that, despite current appearances, this is not who the patient 'really is'. It may be necessary for carers and relatives to understand that although frailty may render the once familiar unrecognizable, the body as identity is unchanged. Sexuality does not depend entirely upon anatomy. Similarly, reassuring an incontinent man that 'it's the disease, not you' makes possible the most intimate of interventions without any loss of dignity: 'when they wash you from head to foot they talk to you. They talk to you all the time and gradually you think "Well, why not?" It's a perfectly natural thing for them to do. All that pride, that silly male pride, gradually it disappears, so you lay back and enjoy it. They do everything with such dignity and care that, in the end, you don't give a damn' (Fred).

Following the principle of a hologram, where every element expresses the whole, de Hennezel (1997: 55) writes 'something of beauty always survives, if only the colour of the eyes.' Judith, however, reached a point where her physical disidentification seemed to indicate feelings of fundamental disintegration. In despair and frustration she groaned 'Oh, my body. I want to get rid of it. It's horrible. My hands both hurt; they're numb. I can't hold things properly. My legs and feet feel peculiar, odd. I have so many problems with rashes and my chest. So many various things go wrong that I just think, "Oh, just get rid of it."' This is a point where tensions between the 'me' that is 'not me', much as for the 'now, but not yet', can become overwhelming. One commonly speaks of being 'beside oneself' in times of acute anxiety and Judith continued 'It's funny, I feel I'm more than one person, especially when they wash you and you're naked. I've had enemas and God knows what, they even have to wipe your bottom. It's awful. I used to hate anyone to see me naked. But it's as if it's happening to somebody else. It's like you're two people, you have to be, or you would never want to speak to the people doing all these terrible things.'

In terminal illness, few dimensions of experience escape some 'renegotiation' (Mathieson and Hendrikus 1995*a*,*b*). One does not have to look far for evidence of ontological disintegration (Giddens 1991). 'Self' can shatter in a multitude of directions. Mary and Carla both described the tensions between their conscious and subconscious readiness for death. Once a keen bridge player, Victor found he could no longer concentrate. Even sound can betray the previously taken for granted. Sadie described herself as sounding 'like an old woman', while Camilla mourned her descent into silence: 'it's a horrible feeling. I know what I sounded like before. You just have to listen to my ansaphone voice. You wouldn't believe it was the same person. It's very, very difficult.' Older people tended to comment most on disparities of intention and ability. Hazel felt she was 'split into two parts. 'Part of me is very old and shaky and not at all good at doing things, but there is part of me that is still alive and can still be of value to someone, to people.' Perhaps because contemporaries were outlived and there was no one with whom to remember the past, Bernard reintroduces themes of marginality and estrangement, describing himself as 'Brain-wise, fine. Body-wise I'm definitely gone. There are a lot of things I would like to do but I can't, I'm not fit enough even to go to a restaurant and have a nice meal, something like that. It's just wishful thinking.'

Regarding herself as 'small and insignificant', Elsie summarizes the experience of self-estrangement: 'I don't feel the same person. I'm not the same person, I feel sad and miserable. I'm not the same person.' Small wonder that in her dreams, so ill at ease, so not at home, she should wander 'round and round, but where I'm going to, and what I'm making for, I can never find out.' Interestingly, in Semitic culture the healed daemonic or divisory impulse is portrayed by a quietly sitting figure. Conventionally clad, self-possessed, the quality of his presence states 'here I am' (with the implication 'and it's alright'). It is not the possession of a religious faith that matters in regard to personal integration, but this deep sense of feeling at home in relation to others and to life generally (Guntrip 1969: 328). As Mary shows, personal relationships, happiness, wholeness and holiness are mutually implicated: 'As an adolescent, I had all sorts of insecurities and feelings of inadequacy. Then, when I became a mother, I moved in a world where people no longer had to be smarter than anybody else. I was just as adequate as anyone else. I enjoyed being a mother. I enjoyed the friends I made. I became involved with a church and I enjoyed what the church gave me. Suddenly, I suppose, I became a whole person and these last 9 years have been the happiest of my life.'

In strange and disorienting situations, symbols of home and safety are particularly cherished. Walking around any women's ward one cannot fail to observe fluffy toys, teddies, dolls and the apparently absurd significance they can hold for some people. Sadie would become quite frantic if her 'Dolly' was ever misplaced: 'Where's my Dolly? Mum and Dad bought it for me. Mum said "I love you. I can't always come up to see you, but I want you to know how much I love you."' The transitional object is perhaps the first symbol encountered in childhood, 'the starting point of our ever elaborating cultural expression of our experience of our environing universe as not de-personalizing us, a world in which 'persons' can feel at home with a sense of belonging' (Guntrip 1969: 330). Symbols, however, are not simply a vehicle for emotion, they have an unlimited capacity for disclosure. When the limits of the 'environing universe' are unspecified, apparently simply requests ('Where's my Dolly?') may carry the gravitas of profound existential enquiry. It is not difficult to find parallels between Sadie's affection for 'Dolly' and the creative endeavours of Tracey's children (Fig. 11.1). Considered with Sadie's repeated 'jokes' about meeting St Peter, it is not unreasonable to wonder whether her longing for 'Dolly' also hints at a convergence of human and ultimate concerns. Certainly, a deep existential note sounded through Sadie's wonderings: 'I want to be angry, but there's nobody to blame for having my life knocked from under me. Before I go to bed, before I go to sleep, I try to say a few things about how I feel … "got us through another day …" and then I think about all the other people who haven't got through. X amount of billions have died today. Why? Why? [voice dropping]. Perhaps there isn't supposed to be a reason, perhaps it's just there.' Dolls frequently act as symbols for a numinous inner self and it is not merely fanciful to hear 'Where am I?' resonating in 'Where is Dolly?' Much as we all say more than we 'know', could Sadie be asking for more than she 'realizes' (in the sense of 'knows' and 'embodies')—expressing needs that extend further than those generally associated with transitional objects? The desire to know oneself and to be able to say 'I am' is bound up with a search for one's place in the ultimate order of things. At its deepest level, 'I am here'—the answer to Sadie's question— is an articulation of spiritual awareness. 'I am here—and it's alright' is our only indication that such yearning has been satisfied. Clearly this was not the case for Sadie.

'Other people don't recognize me'

It has been argued that in the 'broad sweep' of health care provision, women and ethnic minority groups tend to be regarded as 'familiar strangers' (Balarajan 1995). They are construed as 'other' by services arranged in terms of a dominant masculine perspective (Webb 1986). Although a woman's body is more closely associated with grief and death than that of her male counter-part (Bronfen 1992: xi), men receiving palliative care traverse this distance; they invert the norm. Thus, in services shaped by the dominant association of womanhood with death, the vulnerability of these men not only distinguishes them from the masculine ideal, they may also find it is they who are 'other'. Literature on adult grief, for example, tends to be based on studies of women (Hockey 1997: 89) and Williams's (1996) general hospice survey of men and bereavement found that of 36 potential participants, all but four bereaved men could only be contacted through a female relative. The higher female referral rate for this study, coupled with the advanced years of male referrals also implies that carers do not 'see' men in the same way that they 'see' women and that masculinity becomes a less obscuring factor with age. If men are rec-ognized primarily because they are old, they have become Simmel's (1950: 407) strangers of a particular type.

In an ageist society, many of the study participants could be considered 'familiar strangers' simply because of their advanced years. Elsie found 'young people don't come up to me, they seem sort of scared' and Bernard felt that 'when you're old, people sum you up quite differently to how you consider yourself.' Much as an immigrant is a marginal person who, from the vantage point of those he approaches, is without a history (Schutz 1964), old age can bring a similar sense of alienation. Although recollection has the capacity to actualize or remember the past in the here and now (what the ancient Greeks called anemnesis), reminiscence often reveals as much or more about current circumstances (Jonker 1997: 189). When she looked back, Elsie felt as cultural-ly displaced as any migrant: 'Even a simple thing like the telephone, I thought was out of this world, but nobody thinks like that now. We thought it was wonderful, the cat whiskers' crystal radio, where you had to juggle that thing. It might as well be a thousand years away now though, when you talk about it to people.'

Bereavement also becomes a form of exile whose escape is no longer possi-ble in terms of sharing knowledge of events or artefacts, as distinct from infor-mation about them. Even when friends and relations do survive, physical deterioration may render them strangers. After 55 years of marriage, suffering from dementia, Gregory's wife no longer recognized him. Unfortunately, sometimes neither did his carers: 'People might notice that your eyes are not as good, but it does take a long time to get them to realize. I even get people in St Christopher's offering me things, and they've known me for 2 weeks. They say, "Oh look at that ...", but I can't see it. It's a very slow process to get people to understand.' Undoubtedly, this process was impeded when carers noticed the many family photographs decorating Gregory's locker—photographs he could not see, but often held. One is reminded of Chopin, who always carried a small phial of Polish soil, yet died in exile. Sometimes ignored, sometimes overlooked, sometimes the object of condescension, patients were often no longer recognized as before. 'Some people have been great, but a lot of people I've known for years keep away from me. They don't know what to say. It can be very hurtful. I would rather someone came up to me and talked about it than blanked it. You feel like a leper. Maybe they're frightened of catching it. They can't handle it. Men especially keep away until they've had a few drinks, then they get the courage up and they're completely over the top, too affectionate, falling all over you [laughter]' (Jane).

Familiar but different, near yet far, the early hysterical reactions to people with AIDS illustrate the potential of the stranger to provoke communal krisis. Theories of 'mimetic rivalry' (Girard 1986) propose that it is the outsider who is 'most like us' whom we find the most threatening. His proximity to the norm either designates him a source of social change or, like the scapegoat, virtually guarantees his expulsion to the desert. Irene, for example, remained a member of her camping group but 'this summer, unless we went up to them to talk, they seemed to be avoiding me … [sadly and shrugging her shoulders] … Still, there we are, you can't tell what people are like can you?'

In the popular imagination it seems the cancer patient still carries a certain 'contaminating' potential. They are the threatening stranger. One day centre member spoke tearfully of a social event (not at St Christopher's) she had 'really been looking forward to', where she realized that only she was handed a paper cup, not a glass. Contagion is still a powerful metaphor in the social construction of illness (Sontag 1978) and during the course of this research, 'it's not as if it's catching' became a familiar refrain. Tracey explained 'Cancer is like a voodoo thing. Everybody knows that you can't catch it, but they don't like to mix with people who've got it, just in case. They look at you and think "this could be me soon". People shy away from you. They don't really want to have a conversation with you anymore. You hear them whispering "she's got cancer". You hear them talk about you, instead of to you. They exclude you.'

Considering difference in terms of inclusion and exclusion echoes much that has already been said about marginality and health professionals who become patients tend to emphasize the difficulties of migration from one 'side' of the caring relationship to the other (Scannell 1985). Camilla felt her nursing experiences actually made life harder, especially 'coping with other patients, any patients, but especially those like me with MND. I find this really, really difficult. People who are nurses, doctors, they all have the same problem being on the other side of the fence. It's very different and very, very difficult.' Recalling my own startled feelings when a day centre patient asked me 'how long have you been diagnosed?' illustrates the protective function of casting those who are sick as 'other'. Much as confrontational art can bring either delight or pain to the viewer, encountering the existential anguish of another can also be personally deconstructing. As Julia realized 'It's hard to talk about religious or spiritual things without exposing a lot of yourself, and staff might not think that was professional.'

Jane also felt that defensive patterns of relating impede recognition and fail to enlarge restrictive situations, stating 'Having been a nurse, now I'm on the other side, knowing what I know now, I would have been a lot more caring, and showed that I cared. When I took my nurse training, you didn't show any emotions—that was unprofessional. Well, I don't agree with that now. I would sort of show my feelings more. With the patients and the relatives, I'd just be, not more caring, but I'd show that I cared. I'd be more human.' Recognition as a mutuality of giving and receiving, the fullness of humanity realized through plurality-in-unity are statements of spiritual awareness: declarations of the individual's relationship with the whole.

Josie illustrates another schism dividing even the seriously unwell from the terminally ill. Some months after joining the day centre, her problems—although serious—were discovered not to be life threatening. In a traumatizing reversal, where she had once felt most amongst friends, she suddenly became 'other', feeling 'almost guilty that I've survived. It's so strange. It's so hard to change around, I can't—I'm still in shock. I'm choked if I go back to the day centre. Everyone is so pleased for me, but I can't cope with it. I can't speak to them about my feelings any more because, well, they're dying and I'm not. Every time I go back, someone else has gone and I'm still alive. Before, we were a community because we were all in the same boat, but it's not even as if I've had a recovery because I didn't even have cancer.' Clearly, it is not only the absence of a shared past which can render one a stranger, but a divergent future. A discomforting alterity is emphasized by any loss of parity, even a reprieve from impending mortality.

'Treat me normally'

If one function of research is to articulate the views of its subjects, then 'treat me normally' is a major injunction from terminally ill people. Overprotection was often as socially displacing in its consequences as avoidance or rejection. Even on days when her pain was well controlled and she could 'completely forget about it', Eileen's problem was her neighbour: 'she talks me out of things. She sort of turns me off it by saying, "Be careful, don't carry too much, don't do too much." She takes the edge right off it. She smothers me. I mean, she's been a good friend and I wouldn't be without her, but she does keep me in check. I know how far I can go, what I can do. I know my limits.' Similarly, Sadie longed to 'go out, just for an afternoon in a wheelchair, but my husband just won't have any of it. He just won't go with me and it worries him sick if anyone else does. I think he's scared in case anything happens.'

The invocation of 'normality', however, is not a naïve form of denial. Like Hazel, most patients realized that 'People can't treat me the same as before because I'm not the same. I can't get out of doors without someone lifting me into the car or pushing me into the ambulance. It's only logical if people treat me differently.' Rather, 'normality' accommodates special needs whilst recognizing that they occupy less than the whole picture. Personal traits or activities unrelated to illness may be more significant expressions of self. 'Normality' carries an imperative for inclusion that challenges the ambiguity of the stranger. Judith exemplifies the argument thus. Dissimilar, in that she received all her nourishment through a tube directly into her stomach, her universal need for unconditional acceptance and friendship is archetypally expressed: 'Oh, I'd love to be sitting somewhere nice, in a social environment. Drinking from a nicely cut crystal glass. I mean, they can put it straight down the tube into my stomach, but it's just not the same.'

To recognize is to know again, to see the familiar in a new way. In Judith's case this would mean the feeding tube would remain, but its meaning would be altered. Not simply functional, the artificial appliance symbolizes a desire for authentic companionship: the universal need to share our bread. At this level, Judith's story converges with that of the archetypal wanderer, Odysseus. The saga concludes with Odysseus being first recognized, not by Penelope his wife, but by his dog, Argos. For Argos, recognition is instinctive. He sees beyond the obvious because, for him, the obvious—costume, facial hair and the like, are irrelevancies. For Argos, the essential Odysseus is immutable, much as for Eileen, 'smothered' by a neighbour who sees only her infirmities, it is her little dog who will 'go mad when she sees me, run around like crazy, really welcome me back [laughing].' Similarly, the recognition of Judith's feeding tube, with everything this implies about finding ways to help her feel included, invites comparisons with Odysseus' inability to settle until the oar, symbol of his wandering, resembled a winnowing fan—an object not associated with exile.

Estrangement as refuge

Infirmity and the reaction of others may mean that patients feel unrecognizable and unrecognized but, despite their oft-repeated desire for acceptance and inclusion, some people deliberately curtailed their social contacts. As the experience of illness gradually became more consuming, to some degree, this was inevitable. For the seriously ill person, however, self-exposure also carries risks. Anxieties that visitors might dwindle or practical assistance disappear if too many genuine feelings surfaced, were real and frequently expressed. Consequently, people sometimes became 'familiar strangers', conforming to prevailing expectations of 'the sick but brave' by deliberately muting their more dissonant shades of 'otherness'. Judith was not alone in 'putting up a front': 'I try to be reasonably pleasant. People are kind to visit, why should they put up with you sounding off about how rotten life is?' and Mary was careful to nurture her sources of support: 'People have been kind to me—cooked meals, looked after the children, given me lifts, things like that. I try to seem grateful. Otherwise, I think people wouldn't want to help, not if they thought I was getting expectant.'

When friends and family see only infirmity, social encounters affirm the sick person's distance from the norm. Near but far, similar but different, the stranger's situation is inherently stressful. As Charmaz (1983) also noticed in her study of chronically ill people, even as he yearned to be recognized, Bernard entered an apparently 'safe' spiral of withdrawal: 'I want to be with people where you could carry on a conversation like we are now, to be normal, but because my body is not capable I go into myself more.' Hoffmann's experiences as an immigrant are poignant in their similarity: 'The desire for the comfort of being a recognizable somebody placed on a recognizable map breaks in on me with such anguishing force that it scalds my spirit and beats it back into its hiding place'(Hoffman 1989: 140).

If, as Bernard put it, he chose to 'keep up a masquerade', not wanting 'people to see that I am as I am', others also felt it wiser to hide their true feelings. Sometimes the strain became too much to bear. 'You have to put on a brave face but, after a while, it wears thin. Self-pity only pushes people away, then, you're completely on your own. But, as much as I want it not to, the mask does slip. You can't wear it forever. It's not healthy. You have to let things out, release all the tension' (Camilla). Although Sadie went 'out of the way' to appear jovial, she too harboured deep insecurities, many related to her unfamiliar, steroid-induced, shiny round face: 'I feel so cut off. I feel everyone's going "Cor, what's the matter with her?" I do wear blusher and stuff—I copied something in a magazine—and I was beginning to feel quite good. But, as Christmas came nearer and nearer, I began to get more and more in a state. I was worried they'd all have a good look and after I left the room, they'd have a good laugh. Yeah, the mask definitely slips and then you've got tears of a clown, tears of a clown.'

Once forbidden to own land, Jews have been described as 'quintessential strangers' (Madras 1995: 202). Camouflaging his kosher diet as a vegetarian option, Victor illustrates the particular tensions sometimes faced by members of minority groups, reluctant to seem awkward or different: 'I thought it was simpler to say I was vegetarian rather than say I only eat kosher meat. I mean, they might think [said with affected condescension], "Oh, so you're kosher are you? Hey? What's that, then, superior?" No, I don't want to put anyone to any bother.' Although kosher diets are readily available at St Christopher's, Victor was not immediately proffered this option. Given his family history his decision to keep a low profile and take refuge in a vegetarian 'alter ego' are hardly surprising: 'Years ago, there were these pogroms, and my parents had the opportunity of either coming to America, or coming here ... [silence] ... it was all terrible.' Victor's delight when, after a few days, a steward spoke to him in Hebrew and a nurse acknowledged him as Jewish, would seem to indicate a relieved inward shift from the social fringe. This relief was clearly visible in his recounting of the two incidents. Certainly the tension existed, otherwise why should Victor have hesitated to look at the nurse before replying? 'The chap who sells the papers, he looked at me and said, "Shalom". Then, the night before, the male nurse said, "Which restaurant did you work in?" So, I looked at him [pause ... re-enacting a quizzical look], and I said, "Blooms". "Hah", he said, "Salt beef sandwiches!" So, of course, I was feeling at home. He's not Jewish, the nurse, but he said he'd never forget Blooms. His mother was on a coach trip to the Epsom races where they won the sweepstake. On the way back, she said, "I'll treat you, we'll go to Blooms." So, I don't know, it was only a couple of days I'd been here, but I was beginning to feel at home.' Palliative medicine should aspire to an ethos and environment that makes redundant any need for false presentations of self (Goffman 1971), such as that of the Muslim woman who introduced herself as 'Susan—to make things easier.' Perhaps mainstream care could learn from informal or voluntary support groups in this regard. Prior to admission, Victor had sought out such support, 'because if you are left out in the cold, on your own, then you're in trouble.'

Temporal metaphor and making connections

There seems to be something of a coincidence in the reshaping of temporal metaphor and the degree of self-exposure that people settle for. Some patients may have found themselves excluded or voluntarily withdrawing from social contacts, but others remarked on a positive correlation between the friable and dwindling nature of 'their' time and a new-found potential for connecting with others. Eileen found she could 'talk to people more than I would have done before. Whereas someone would have to talk to me before I would talk to them, now I can go up and talk to people.' Jane felt that because the thought of dying was always subconsciously present, 'You bypass all the niceties and you are bound together quicker, because you know you haven't got a lot of time. If you get on well with someone, you try and cram everything in, because you know that time isn't on your side.'

Compared with other patient groups, the speed with which some terminally ill patients are able to enter the therapeutic process has not gone unnoticed: 'it seems that under the pressures of a life and death situation, untapped sources are activated and expressed' (Bach 1990: 9). When emotional depths are traversed at speed, however, patients are vulnerable, not only to the inappropriate transference of emotion but, given that their peers will also die shortly, to the pains of multiple bereavement. Whether temporary or long term, refuge could be found in a voluntary estrangement. Jane, for instance, was 'Normally guarded before I get to know someone, but it happens so quick now. Lately though, I try not to get too friendly when new people come to the day centre. You know they're just gonna go. It's painful. I shall probably go back there, make new friends, and get hurt again. I try to get used to it, but the last one knocked me silly. I was really looking forward to seeing Betsy. I had a present and everything for her. When I asked where she was, they looked at me a bit strange and said she was dead. That really brings it home. There's only me and Daniel left now out of our little group ... who's gonna be the next one, him or me?'

Social withdrawal is clearly a more complex matter than simply feeling unrecognized, or not wishing to reveal aspects of one's self. Other patients 'further down the road' embody one's own inevitable deterioration in ways that can be difficult to face. Camilla particularly found mixing with other patients a trial: 'if I go down to physiotherapy and there's somebody else there, I just ignore them. It's as if they don't exist. It's not me, it's not them, really it's staring reality in the face, and it ain't much fun. So, I tend to keep myself aside and not to see any one.' Even so, withdrawal and introspection should not automatically be interpreted as signs of depression and despair (although they could be). If liminality increasingly becomes their metier and conventional temporality feels increasingly alien, some people may actually want to explore or quietly reflect on their 'otherness'. Just as clearing away Hazel's dead flowers, reminding her to 'let go', would have deprived her of their spiritual support, the desire to occupy or distract patients, so emphasizing their 'normality', may not always be appropriate. Remembering that it is the still point of the fulcrum that permits movement, some patients may need to experience the inner siftings of silence if they are to face the unknown with any degree of equanimity.

If carers feel uneasy with such patients, their agitation should act as a clarion prompting them to examine their own motivation and anxieties. It is easier to encourage patients to 'do' things than to share some of the uncertainties that stillness may reveal. The carer's prototypical 'Can I get you anything?' also maintains the inherent inequalities of a subject–object pattern of relating. Reducing carer–patient duality, 'What do you need?' has a wider, less focused orbit. Certainly, the unpredictable response carries greater risks for carers, but it is more likely to be meaningful. As auxiliary nurse, I asked Joan whether I could fetch her anything. She replied 'No, I'm fine, thank you.' Only minutes later, when I asked what she might need, tears welled: 'Comfort, only comfort.' This brings us to a difficult paradox. Unless 'otherness' is accommodated— Joan as a person, for whom, beyond a certain level, 'things' were virtually use-less—there can be no genuine contact. Such accommodation, however, is underwritten by a fundamental unity. We are all people for whom 'things' can lose their meaning, relative to the universal need for love.

Health/whole: inevitable synonym?

Thus far, the stranger has been considered only as a mediator and illuminator of illness. His denouement, however, can also express a dawning realization of one's previous self-estrangement or unconscious estrangement from others. Only when he became ill did Claude consider whether the 'main thing' he needed to do was to 'try and find out my wife's feelings, instead of imagining what they might be. I can only do that by talking to her. It's hard when you've lived together for 30-odd years, because I've always been rather quiet and never discussed anything. It's hard to start, risking a rebuff, perhaps for articu-lating some imagined view of the other person, and then finding you've got it completely wrong.'

Sometimes suffering exposes the inaccuracies of one's previously assumed identity. Viewed retrospectively, through the lens of serious illness, missed brush strokes, smudges and flaws can be seen in the once 'accurate' self-portrait. From the vantage point of old age, for instance, Hazel could see that she 'dodged about from one thing to another. I didn't connect with people. Really, I was frozen for most of my life. I've been looking at some photos of myself and I'm amazed. I was really very good looking, but I didn't know or realize. I didn't see myself in that light at all.' Similarly, on becoming ill, it was the love and attention Julia received from others that prompted her radical self-re-orientation. 'It was only when I got cancer that I got all the niceness and kindness that people usually wait until you're dead to say. For the first time in my life I realized that people actually liked me. Before, I valued myself so little that unless I was district manager, I was nothing. Suddenly, I didn't need to work in that obsessive way any more. Although I shrank physically about 2 inches, mentally, I went down about 6 feet. There are people who look at me now and say, "Were you always that small?" because when I was at work with all that power and dominance I was 6 feet high and 6 feet wide—people got out of my way when I walked down the corridor. Now I have to assume that body language to get people jumping and I feel sick and disgusted with myself when I do it. It was a suit of armour I wore when I was an inadequate person. Now, after all that has happened, I have a much more realistic idea of my size and I don't feel sorry or ashamed or inadequate to the same extent. Of course, there are a lot of things I can't do now, but I don't want to be anything but myself.' Julia's experience brings to mind the stranger as *xenos* where, in a process of liberating disillusionment, processes of knowing and becoming are realized. Without wishing to 'gloss over' the traumas of estrangement and terminal illness, there is something here of coming home, of viewing oneself from another place and becoming aware, not only of the myopia and distortions of earlier perceptions (what a stranger one was to oneself), but also their restrictive implications.

Were Julia's insights to be located in our prism, they might be found where 'letting go' (that is, of her once taken-for-granted persona) intersects with the stranger: stranger as *xenos*, and the stranger who bears gifts. Similarly, given her total paralysis, Carol's unique and startling proclamation 'I am me at last, free to be my own silly self.' Neither woman 'worked out' the self-appreciation that enabled her to live in a new way, but their experiences disclose paradoxes of finding in losing, of potential in a time of loss. Perhaps this is what Edinger (1973: 163) means when he writes 'Man must be parted from that on which he is dependent but which he is not, before he can become that which he is, unique and indivisible.'

In this sense, 'I am' (May *et al.* 1950: 43) may be an utterance made by few, but the desire for the authenticity it expresses is not uncommon. Personal growth is sometimes instinctively considered in terms of a distancing or estrangement from the familiar—echoing Augustine on the widow as one who is free to explore her understanding of ultimate issues. Tracey seems to concur: 'It's hard to make yourself someone else, to pour yourself out. It would be easier if the kids were grown up, then you could take the time to find yourself.' Self-knowledge resulting from estrangement evokes Hebraic connotations of gift. Our concern nevertheless remains the range of existential commitment implied in such a notion, whether we are dealing with anything ultimately or spiritually significant.

Stranger bearing gifts

From a sociological perspective, the idea of the stranger as one bearing gifts is not novel (Simmel 1950). Endowed with a certain 'objectivity' by his refocusing pattern of near and farness, the stranger can be uniquely perceptive and receptive. Bringing a 'fresh eye' to situations, he frequently receives confidences that might be withheld from someone more closely related. Perceiving an interviewer as stranger may make it easier for patients to talk. Certainly, interviews sometimes have unpredictable pay-offs. Tracey used hers to display her mothering skills, Edwin shared a dark secret, Arthur pressed his case for remaining in the hospice. 'Otherness' also invites speculation and startling projections—such as Carla's view of myself as a 'beautiful specialist in tragedy'.

Allowing herself to cry only with someone from outside her family, Tracey demonstrates how, in offering relief without responsibility, the stranger may provide a safety and discretion unavailable elsewhere. Josie, for example, would 'ring the Samaritans when I was depressed. It's nice to talk to someone who doesn't know you, who you feel isn't judging you. I feel comfortable off-loading to them. My mum just denies everything, I can't talk to her because my feelings might devastate her.' Stiles's (1990) qualitative study of nurse–family relationships likens the contributions of home care nurses to that of a 'shining stranger'—a personification derived from family comments about the nurses. The skills, contacts and information offered by professionals may be entitlements, but the appreciation they solicit suggests they can feel like gifts. Victor could not speak too highly of those caring for him: 'They put their heart and soul into it, over and above what they need to do. Their professionalism is wonderful.' The effects of a high staff–patient ratio were often interpreted in terms of the 'specialness' of carers. In Jane's words, 'It's so different to hospital here. If I have to keep ringing the bell the nurses just say, "Don't worry, that's what we're here for." Nothing's too much trouble. Any other nurse would think, "blooming nuisance."' To regard any 'gift relationship' as exclusively one way, however, is unwise. The processes of recognition implied in coming to know a stranger can carry benefits for all parties. Stiles's home care nurses, for example, learned as much as they shared: 'There are those patients, who, without being aware of it, also take care of the people who take care of them' (de Hennezel 1997: 3).

Recurrent images of masks, the clown or the joker, may convey a patient's feelings of exclusion, but they can also endorse the perceptiveness of their observations. The seer is as likely as the 'fool' to appear in costume. Indeed they may be one and the same person. Despite his apparent clumsiness, the clown understands love, sorrow, fidelity; the critical stuff of life. His liberating perspective makes boundary situations tolerable, with laughter creating emotional space and acting as a 'signal of transcendence' (Berger 1997). As an 'amateur' in a professional milieu, it is his 'ordinariness', his 'innocence' (as distinct from any gullibility) that allows the clown to exercise originality and creativity, bringing home the lesson that it is not always what one does, but who one is, that matters to the 'recipient' (Faber 1971).

The stranger can offer perceptive insights, impartial judgements and novel practical ability. From the perspective of depth psychology, however, his 'gift' is the possibility for personal wholeness and a meaningful integration of disowned, denied or projected aspects of the self. The critical issue for anyone concerned with meeting spiritual needs, however, remains the existential remit of the 'whole person', in this instance, whether patients' reflections on and experiences of estrangement draw attention to a spiritual dimension of personhood, or to any ultimate significance in the human story. To explore the success of psychological, sociological or other narratives in accommodating the range and depth of human experience we turn to Carla and Edwin, both of whom demonstrate the powerful and mediating influence of 'the stranger' for people who are terminally ill.

Carla's bride

Always a prodigious artist, it was surprising to enter Carla's room and find her knitting a white shawl. For one whose sartorial preferences tended to range from pale lilac to deep purple, her white dress was also unusual. Smiling and relaxed, she announced 'I think I've finished with painting. I've no more pictures left in me now.' Virtually her final work, her distinctively bridal Fig. 12.2 was completed only days before she died: 'I don't know why I did this, it just sort of came out.' Although never referred to as a self-portrait, does any work fail to expose some aspects of its creator's identity, articulate something of the inner life? There is a passing resemblance in the high forehead and centre parting of the hair but it is the symbolisms of this work that invite speculation.

Neither maid nor wife, the bride is a quintessentially liminal figure and the symbolic wedding or marriage appears frequently in thanatology (Wheelwright 1981: 98, 181). Common embarrassing slips of the tongue where wedding is uttered for funeral or vice versa, film titles such as *Brides of Dracula* or *Four weddings and a funeral* expose the subconscious association of union, new beginnings and death. In view of her situation, therefore, Carla's subject is entirely appropriate. The insubstantial and ungrounded lower body and the pink and red colouring connote the fading and gathering in of life, calling to mind the last sheaves of harvest. Always carried in by a woman, the final sheaf was once decorated with red ribbons, calling to mind the blood sacrifice of more ancient harvest rituals (Rees 1992: 32). The trinitarian buttons suggest dynamics of thesis, antithesis, synthesis—movement towards a new state of being, also invoking the classical tripartite sense of destiny:

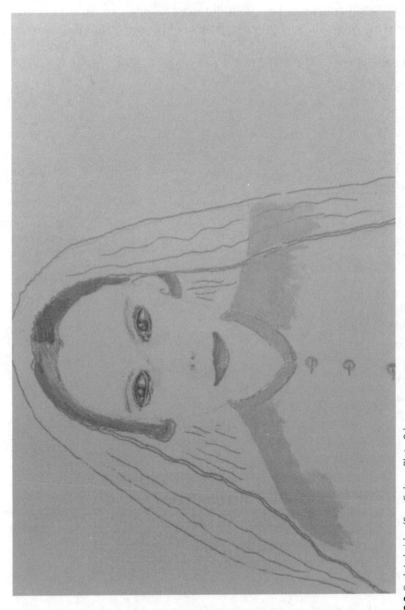

Figure 12.2 Carla's bride. (See Colour Plate 9.)

Clotho spins, Lachesis measures and Atropo cuts the cloth of life. The unfurrowed brow and enigmatic smile, however, intimate contentment and a secret source of strength. How this somewhat ethereal image could result from one so physically tethered by her hugely distended abdomen, cough and fractured leg, is a mystery. Although only days from death, demonstrating that the trans-rational is not always trans-experiential, Carla was nevertheless pleased with her new clothes and cheerful that she no longer needed to paint. If it is true that 'consciousness is not a given but a task' (Ricoeur 1974: 328), then the symbolism of Fig. 12.2 endorses Carla's instinctive understanding. Her 'task' of painting had drawn to a close. Using a term borrowed from alchemy, the transparency of the image, its white and gold, indicate a 'transmutation' where intimacy and union matter more than productivity.

The bride is an archetypal image invoking notions of Coniunctio (Wheelwright 1981: 280), the coming together of opposites and the marital union symbolizes psychological transformation or wholeness (Leonard 1987; Woodman 1985). Fairy tales contain abundant examples of opposing rifts and their eventual healing. The story of the marriage of Beauty and the Beast, for instance, may be read as the healing of a damaging schism between man's higher and his animal self. This schism is harmful because, separated from Beauty and all she symbolizes, her father dies and the Beast, very nearly (Bettelheim 1991: 308–9). By the time she does marry, however, Beauty no longer regards her sexuality as repulsive or animal like. The 'shadow' has been accepted and her love for her father and the Beast are not opposed. The route to 'happy ever after' lies wide open. Beauty's virginity is less a description of sexual experience than a metaphor for developing personal integrity. Indeed, the original meaning of virgin is to be 'one-in-herself' (Harding 1955: 125). But what is the degree of existential commitment subsiding in terms such as 'personal integrity' or 'one-in-herself'? Given the symbolisms of Carla's painting, it is entirely reasonable to ponder whether it manifests an irreducible and ultimate dimension of human experience.

The case for a spiritual interpretation

With her combined sensuality and demure aspect, Carla's bride is a modern representation of an ancient understanding pre-dating any contemporary psychological viewpoint. Her image recalls the composure typical of the healed daemonic impulse. It echoes, therefore, an understanding of the whole person as one whose thoughts and actions are infused with a meaning whose genesis lies beyond human creativity. The transcendent life, however, is not reached in some remote and abstract realm but in daily acts of living. Every moment, regardless of its outcome, is charged with an ultimate significance, wherein lies human contentment. Perhaps this explains Carla's satisfaction with her knitting, which she freely admitted was unlikely to reach completion.

Something of that experience which May (1950: 43) describes as a sense of the ultimate rightness and unity of personal existence typifies significant acts or moments. There is a quality and assurance of presence which, again in Hebraic thought, would indicate not simply that 'I am', but that 'I am ready'. Generally such moments of prescience do not result from personal endeavour. They are experienced as a gift. From this perspective, it is small wonder that Carla's picture 'just came' to her. Interestingly, in many cultures brides wear red and white is worn to funerals. Their combination in an image produced by one so close to death possibly indicates a certain degree of preparation, compliance and readiness for the inevitable. For one so oppressed by physical necessity, sometimes sharing her deep sorrow at leaving her family, to interpret the calmness of Carla's last days simply as denial seems a spurious and reactive closure of possibility. There is a nagging sense in which the psychological explanation of such a 'gift', exclusively in terms of inner union, occludes a wider vision.

Brides and marriage have long, and universally, been associated with cosmic consciousness and our sense of the transcendent. In Greek mythology, creative fulfilment is represented by the marriage of Dionysus to Ariadne; Danae, indicating the sacred life-giving marriage of heaven and earth, was impregnated by Zeus in the form of a golden shower; Roman notions of the sun and moon as an eternally dancing bridal brother and sister resonate in the words of St Ambrose, 'the creator has granted this bridal sister-star of the sun the power of showing forth the mystery of Christ' (Rahner 1963: 159, 164); and a native American prayer chant begins:

> O mother earth and father sky,
> Your children are we, and with tired backs
> We bring you the gifts you love.
> Then weave for us a garment of brightness.
> O mother earth and father sky.
> (Astrov 1962: 221)

The grounds for arguing that Carla's contentment—her painting is but its expression—results from some spiritual or ultimate sense of meaning, are at least as solid as those whereon the claims of depth psychology are staked. The two approaches, however, do not exist in simplistic opposition. Addressing the same material, the critical issue is which most thoroughly exhausts its disclosive potential. The existence of a horizon beyond that broached by psychology in no sense 'disproves' the foreground, but the wider angle does alter its meaning, depriving psyche of the final word. For these reasons alone, the bridal image merits further examination.

In Carla's depiction, the unblemished open countenance reminds us of the head as a traditional seat of divine power, of Sahsrara the seventh chakra, the entry point for the human life-force, pouring from the wider universe or a divine source, of Pentecost and the tongues of flame. Although the veil indicates respect and rites of passage, masking or covering the body can also represent possession in terms of feeling claimed or cherished. The prophet Elijah, for example, called Elisha to be his disciple by throwing his cloak over him (*Kings* Chapter 19, Verses 19–21). Commenting on certain recurring colours in the dreams of a terminally ill client, 'Gold is the highest colour value and may be likened to the sun. White refers to consciousness', Wheelwright (1981: 56) is encouraged by their indication of enlarged personal consciousness and an advanced point of psychic integration. Many spiritual traditions, however, would wish to augment this interpretation. Christ's transfiguration—'His face shone like the sun, and his clothes became as white as the light' (*Matthew* Chapter 17, Verse 2)—affirmed his supernatural identity. Golden images of the Buddha indicate his enlightenment. Perhaps the iridescent lips, head, ears and eyes of Carla's bride (interestingly, all sites used in the anointing of the sick) affirm some realization on her part of Tillich's ontological philosophy of religion (Tillich 1964b), where religion points to and expresses an infinite and spiritual dimension that is rooted in the structure of being itself. Certainly, the transmutation of base material into gold has long operated as a metaphor for spiritual growth, and the shining eyes of Fig. 12.2 invite comparison with the female Japanese shamans of Yamashiro. Invariably blind, and so without distraction, these women are considered to possess heightened 'inner' sight, or extra-ordinary powers of discernment (Rees 1992: 112). As Rees notes; elsewhere, these shamans are called brides: in Ethiopia the novice is assigned two 'best men' should her spiritual husband present her with any problems (Lewis 1971: 57–63). In the voodoo cults of Haiti, women may enter a spiritual marriage receiving both a certificate and ring (Metraux 1959: 215).

Christ's extraordinary capacity to affect transformation was revealed at a marriage feast and the Old Testament *Song of songs*, depicting the relationship of the bridegroom and his beloved, has long served as a metaphor of the spiritual life. For St Bernard, St Victor, St Theresa, John of the Cross and innumerable others it was inevitable and natural for human marriage to provide the best image of the 'fulfilment of life' and Perfect Love (Underhill 1995: 136). As the Haitian and Japanese shamans indicate, however, a 'spiritual marriage' is not confined to the Christian tradition and the seven mystical stages of the Sufi may begin in adoration, but they too end in spiritual union.

This discussion of the symbolic potential of Carla's painting lies within a wider consideration of the phenomenon of the stranger. What has been at stake, and repeatedly emphasized, is the existential commitment implied in any gift the stranger may bear. From the psychological perspective, the bride suggests that personal unity and a broadened state of consciousness result from integrating one's inner 'strangers'. Whilst this may be so, the theological and spiritual implications of this symbol may not simply be swept aside. The peace and purposefulness from which Carla's image emerged are precious gifts whose ultimate dimension also demands recognition.

Edwin's dilemma

Edwin's story also illustrates how metaphors of estrangement mediate personal identity and exposes the existential potential of human relationships. The events of his troubled life, coalescing in terms of an apparently fundamental dilemma, demonstrate how sociological and psychological factors can bring individuals to points of ultimate or theological exploration. Edwin's is the story of the 'unfinished man', the man searching for 'the courage to accept oneself as accepted in spite of being unacceptable' (Tillich 1962: 160). Intuitively recognizing that 'the past is myself' (Bielenberg 1984), he is the man struggling with whether this is exhaustively so. In short, Edwin raises issues concerned with the compatibility of compassion and justice, with sources of meaning when life seems devoid of an ultimate dimension and with how far a man's actions constitute his identity and personal 'worth'. All these issues fall within the aegis of the stranger for they address tensions of self and non-self and life's potential for gift—both in terms of encounter and 'forgiveness'.

The outsider

Softly spoken and slightly withdrawn, Edwin presented as an 'outsider'. He recounted his life in terms of a gradual drift towards the fringe. Painfully different from childhood peers because he was dyslexic ('If I was asked to stand and read, I'd go red as a beetroot, I couldn't. It was so embarrassing') and, as an adult, from civilian life and even his family, Edwin eventually found himself living in a foreign land. 'A year after I left the army, I split with me wife. It happens to a lot of service people; civilian life is so different. In the army everything is done for you. Outside, I didn't earn much, and I'd got to find the rent, shoes for the kids—I had five kids. I was going, "I ain't got the money", but my wife, she couldn't see that. I started to drink. I was thieving and I went to prison. Anyway, I thought, "I gotta get outa this", so I joined the French Legion. To me, it was a new start, and we were sent to a state in Africa.'

Although occurring some years later, the tardy diagnosis of Edwin's illness further develops themes of exclusion and non-recognition: 'It was a vicious circle of pain killers and constipation tablets. Round and round I kept going to the doctor, but basically not one of them examined me, not one of them— even though for 6–8 months I'd been lying on me side because I couldn't sit down. I was angry. I still am. If only the doctor had taken more time months ago, I might not be in this situation now. When I talk about it, I feel like bawling me eyes out. It's like a dream, a soap opera, but it ain't no dream. I'd been at the hospital only 10 weeks previous, so I had a go at the doctor I saw then. He just shrugged his shoulders and said, "these things happen."' This failure to recognize and meet Edwin's individual needs hallmarked virtually all his early care. Echoing earlier classroom humiliations, even the gauche breaking of his diagnosis ensured his illness became a 'spectacle' for others: 'He could of told me better. The doctors were all around the bed, and I think it's a personal thing. He should have said, "I'll come back and see you later", instead of everybody around, everyone could hear.'

The following crisis was the first in a rapid and alarming 3 weeks that culminated in Edwin's hospice admission. Metaphors of control are easily detected. 'A soft lump came up on me back and me doctor sent me to hospital straightaway. I couldn't breath and I didn't know what was going on. Things was all happening too fast, everything was wrong. I went to wash meself, but all the faeces come away in me hand. The faeces couldn't come out because of this cancer in the way, so it burrowed up through me skin to make another channel. No wonder I was in pain.'

Once Edwin realized 'the very most I've got is months, not years', he seemed to vacillate between feelings of compromised masculinity, 'I was talking to the workmen, but my partner, she just took over' and an attitude of heroic resistance, 'Just to get more time you've got to fight it and believe you can beat it, or you might as well give in.' Although these extremes suggest a painful sense of personal dislocation, Edwin was more troubled by memories of a certain tragic incident. He seemed almost to regard this event as the 'defining moment' of his life. Certainly, its contemplation constituted an existential crisis, bringing into stark relief his most painful experience of exclusion, his inability to feel any kind of what he called 'spiritual connection'. 'I've tried, you know, praying, but nothing's happened. And I've thought, "this is a load of rubbish. He's supposed to talk to me, to give me a sign or something." They've been very good to me, the churches, so I can't run them down. I've been to the Catholic service, at the time for me own ends, but what have I got at the end of it?' Sighing and sounding very sad, he continued 'It's a funny subject. I think to be religious you have to be brought up in it, and I never was. Perhaps I'm looking at it the wrong way because I don't understand this prayer business. It's such a complicated thing. Perhaps in me heart I hope it's true, but in me mind, I can't grasp it.'

It would be hard to find a neater apologia combining magical thinking (Rozin *et al.* 1986) with the stranger's lot and the missed opportunity that renders one forever spectator, never participant. Even so, the man who sometimes pondered whether Jesus was a spaceman continued to yearn 'The nearer you get to that point [that is, death], I think your views might change. Everybody wants something to grasp on, everybody wants it.'

Nihilism or punishment?

Analogies between the emergence of Edwin's troubling story and his fistula painfully burrowing to the surface, are tempting. As much as any organic development, guilt can infiltrate the 'fabric' of personhood, striking at the very heart of tensions of self and non-self, so inflicting a profound ontological claustrophobia. As Levinas (Llewelyn 1995: 18) explains, 'The sharpness of shame derives from a conjunction of not being able to understand how one could have done such a thing and not being able to deny one's identity with the being who did it ... Adam was naked and he hid himself, but even if he could hide himself from Eve or God, he could not hide his nakedness from himself ... nakedness is not being unclothed. It is the need of an apologia for one's existence. It is not motivated by the sense of having done something wrong. It is not conditioned by one's being finite. It is the condition of one's being.'

To be naked is to be vulnerable. Consequently, the depth of Edwin's despair is indicated by his decision to talk, for the first time in his life, about events that occurred when he was stationed in Africa. Perhaps obliquely 'testing the water', a general statement concerning the problem of suffering and a fairly heavy narrative cue preceded his story: 'I can't believe there's a God who's so good that he lets a load of kids die, or wars. I mean I don't believe in wars any more. I think it's a stupid thing and I would never do it again, I wouldn't.' Although, strictly speaking, if one does not believe in God (or rather, a loving God), the classic 'problem of evil' does not exist. Edwin's preoccupations and tortured ambivalence display the strain of one who perceives 'the absence of God and the unchecked power of evil in the world, [so that] it seems there is no God, yet when one feels oneself obsessed with this absence and power, on the other hand, it seems there is no escape from God" (Dunne 1983: 52). As Edwin said 'I want to believe in God, but I reject it. I wouldn't say I'm an atheist, a part of me wants to believe, but there's something like the devil saying, "No you don't want to believe that." It's like a pair of scales, one pulling on the other. Most people, when they come to the end, they're trying to put theirself right. I'm in between whether I do or I don't believe.'

As the interview progressed, Edwin's voice dropped to a whisper, the atmosphere grew fragile and the universal problem tentatively assumed the dimensions of his own specific anguish. The microphone was fastened to his dressing gown so that, on playback, his increasingly loud heartbeat was clearly audible. 'When we were sent to this state in Africa, the orders was "you shoot them", because there was rebels there. When you go into a situation like that, no one can say they're not frightened, you're bloody frightened. Keep yourself alive, never mind them, they're nothing. I had people dropping their guns, coming out, putting their hands up, and I had to shoot them. At the time, I thought nothing of it. It wasn't a problem doing this and I've done other things too, similar to this. But about 7 or 8 years ago, I started thinking about it, mainly at night. I'll start sweating. You can see it, everything you've done. I wake up shouting, going through the jumping out the aeroplanes. You don't exactly think it, you visualize it. It's still there. I'm not proud of myself I can tell you, not proud at all ... but ... [voice fading] it's what I done.'

Much here resonates with the experience of post-traumatic stress disorder. Edwin may have been reassured to learn that his symptoms were far from uncommon and to have discussed them with an expert (Eichelman 1985; Glover 1984). The stranger who discovers himself through and with another, or discovers that he has peers (for strangers are always strangers of a particular type), may no longer be understood exclusively in terms of *extraneous*. There is a potential for *xenos* to emerge as he hears of how others have dealt with experiences similar to his own. Such may have been the case for Edwin. Certainly, the guilty veteran's search for meaning (Thomas 1996: 13) is not unique, neither is the constraint of the individual conscience by institutional demands: 'In the army you're taught to do something. You have to do it. You might not want to, but you do' (Edwin).

In telling his story Edwin becomes Levinas' naked man, the man with nowhere to hide. Returning to the *Genesis* narrative, however, when God entered the Garden he did not call 'What have you done?' but 'Adam, wherefore art thou?' This is surely an invitation easily transposed into a primary objective of modern palliative care. Patients should feel able to say 'Here I am', not in terms of location, but of identity. To search for a meaningful life is to search for unconditional acceptance (Dunne 1975: 37) and given that the search for meaning is one aspect of human spirituality, the safety wherein such exposures become possible is inextricably bound with the provision of spiritual care. Nevertheless, Edwin's imagery—the scales of justice, his naive personification of evil—betray his commitment to the necessarily transparent 'moral economy' of childish or immature reasoning, so that he now regarded himself as 'in the position of what I've done to other people. Alright, they died there and then, but I'm in a position where I'm gonna go the same way but I'm really gonna suffer. It won't be the same as on the spur of the moment. I am being punished for what I done.'

Although Edwin yearned for that 'encounter with the unknown … that seems to underlie the great religions' (Dunne 1975: 86), its possibility was also his major source of anxiety. For Edwin, a defining characteristic of God is deliverance of the just verdict and Edwin felt his wartime actions merited punishment. When the ultimate expression of concern is a justice or 'old order' reckoning (Dunne 1975: 37) that connects actions with consequences in a symmetrical 'tit' for 'tat', dread is an inevitable consequence. Those who find themselves 'naked', are tormented by a fear that makes it impossible for them to 'safely' die (Kierkegaard 1968: 150). Although an apparently less dangerous option lies in denying any ultimate patterning in life's events, this may exact the price of nihilism so that, as Edwin found, life becomes meaningless: 'When you go, that's it. Umph, down in that hole. But, if that's all it is, well what's the purpose of all this? What's the point of being here?'

Nihilism or gift?

By introducing concepts of purpose and meaning, Edwin's dilemma—nihilism or punishment, effects a shift of emphasis. Albeit as a tacit concern, the dilemma's 'flip' side demands attention. Although framed inversely as a conflict between justice and forgiveness, Edwin's preoccupation explores and challenges life's existential potential for gift. That is, the degree to which outcome may exceed expectation, both in terms of human relationships and ultimate encounter (although this is a somewhat false dichotomy for other than in immediate circumstances we have nowhere else to search for the dilemma's solution). For the concept of gift to lead back to metaphors of estrangement frequently occurs in discussions of otherness. At least one literary forerunner exists in Camus's L'Etranger (1981). If Christ is the archetypal stranger ('the world knew him not' (John Chapter 1, Verse 10)), Camus's main character, Meurseult, is his alter ego, the 'outsider' who manifests the world's 'benign indifference'. The truth does not set one free and Meurseult is the man who gives nothing and who knows, ultimately, that nothing will be given. Although a detailed exposition lies beyond these confines, similar polarities are easily flagged up in philosophy. Heidegger, for instance, denies transcendence in the sense of Being beyond the world and, despite addressing himself to the reader, insists the other can give me nothing of importance. Alternatively, Levinas calls to mind aspects of Buber's 'I and Thou' where human existence is not something simply 'to hand' but is received as 'gift'. Levinas presents an ethical face-to-face relationship with the Other which, while individual and contingent, is simultaneously transcendent. That is, the Other comes from 'outside' without mediation, as an ethical injunction or command inscribed on the face of any other person. It might seem that otherness cannot be theoretically addressed without, in some way, reducing its alterity, that which makes it other, but Levinas argues face manifests the Infinite, in a way that is not thematizable. Thus, 'God' may avail himself to human senses, but 'he' cannot be captured by words or thought. The primary spiritual experience, therefore, is always the most authentic. Second-order propositions or talks about God, as Edwin knew only too well, are ultimately unsatisfactory.

Of course, both Heidegger and Levinas have each attracted criticism (Kemp 1996). When considering Edwin's dilemma, however, what matters is that unless one ventures into explicitly theological territory it seems there is no possibility of solving ultimate problematics. Crucial metaphysical disputes and their resolutions are grounded not in abstraction but experience and this is exactly the criterion on which philosophy (and many other disciplines) disappoints. As Wittgenstein (1979: 3e) writes, 'For someone broken up by love an explanatory hypothesis won't help much—it will not bring peace.' Clearly, when considering the depths of meaning subsiding in patients' metaphors of estrangement, some approach in addition to philosophical inquiry is required. Edwin reveals a yearning deeper than the purely intellectual. He exposes humanity's need for the caress or presence that, without articulating 'answers', brings a consolation that deprives existential crises of their sting.

Enlarging the picture: hearing the tacit

At its deepest point, Edwin's dilemma may be interpreted as his desire to understand the connection between an action and its consequences. As such, it is both a quest for wisdom and its expression. In the Judaeo-Christian tradition, which is where Edwin locates himself, wisdom symbolizes an awareness of life's ultimate design and purpose. Wisdom suggests ways of living that bring contentment and harmonious relations, but also has the capacity to surprise and subvert conventional expectations. This can sometimes invoke an ambivalent response, including that of fear: 'Moral failure from Wisdom's perspective, is not the result of resistance to an authoritative teacher or text, but unwillingness to read the signs of the times and to discern the processes that make for life and for death for ourselves and our communities' (O'Connell Killen 1997: 12).

Had Edwin come to recognize his own wisdom, rather than hoping for revelations from some distant source, perhaps some of his discomfort could have been reduced. Unfortunately, however, his chronically low self-esteem—in the space of an hour he shamefully announced his lack of education, abandonment of his family, drinking problem, numerous convictions, violent temper and war crimes—effectively eclipsed any positive self-awareness. Nevertheless, Edwin displayed qualities which may be regarded both as a demonstration and product of the wisdom he actually desired. He was, for instance, deeply preoccupied with the concept of justice and his distinctions of head from heart reveal a preference for experiential or authentic knowledge over information. Similarly, he displayed a keen regard for truth, urging his doctor to 'talk straight, I want to know what the score is.'

Concern and affection for his current partner and her family also surfaced: 'Edie must feel just as bad as I do.' These positive attributes, however, remained tacit insofar as they were present, but unrecognized. Approached from this angle, the polarities of Edwin's dilemma begin to crumble. The fundamental issue becomes not a choice between two abstractions, but one of personhood. The dilemma addresses processes of self-recognition and self-discovery where, as always, the critical issue is the existential implication of any process of becoming. Possibly Edwin's desire to 'sort meself out, before it's too late', coupled with his frustrated yearning for ultimate meaning, indicates a shift of identity—from the *extraneous* stranger to *xenos*, from a marginal to a liminal status. Might it not be that any 'waiting is itself the beginning. Who is it that is waiting on the new man ... is it not the new man waiting to come forth? It begins to appear that the man who is dissatisfied is himself the new man ... and has been there all along. His waiting on the new man is a waiting on himself; it is the new man's waiting to come forth. His coming then is a realization in the double sense of that word, a coming to know and a coming to be' (Dunne 1983: 98).

Paradoxically, each of us can 'know more than we can tell and we can tell nothing without relying on our awareness of things we may not be able to tell' (Polanyi 1958: x). Edwin was tacitly aware of more about 'this prayer business', than he could articulate for, 'Waiting on the unknown amounts to waiting on this man within the man, it seems waiting for him to come forth. Waiting is like praying, and insight when it comes, is like the answer to prayer' (Dunne 1983: 96).

Dunne's depiction of 'old' and 'new' men veers uncomfortably towards an image of Russian dolls stacked one within the other, as distinct from a dimensional and more inclusive vision of personhood. Nevertheless, the overall thrust remains: 'we have a principle other than self within us' (Harper 1966: 45). Far from the spiritually moribund creature he considers himself, Edwin's longings may be interpreted as a demonstration of this principle. Despite his primitive imagery of the scales and the pulling devil, his yearning for spiritual experience tacitly suggests that 'the whole man is not a balance of opposing powers, the creative and the destructive powers of the flesh balanced together against the controlling power of the spirit. He is led by another power altogether, a power that has its own goal and its own way, a power that leads him out of his withdrawal and solitude into an entirely new adventure' (Dunne 1983: 100).

Were these issues considered with a skilled and gentle spiritual director, perhaps Edwin's dilemma would have seemed less constricting. He may have come to possess his own 'signs' of spiritual awareness, to realize that they were simply of an unexpected order and that his earlier non-recognition located him firmly in the tradition to which he aspired—much as Mary Magdalene mistook Christ for a gardener and the disciples failed to recognize him on the road to Emmaus. Similarly, by learning to cherish his desire for authentic understanding (rather than experiencing it as a cause for despair), perhaps Edwin would have realized that finding a solution to his 'dilemma' was not entirely his own responsibility. He was not responsible for creating a belief for himself in the way one learns a magic trick. All that was required of him was the attitude he already held, one of non-closure, a refusal to completely rule out the possibility of ultimate meaning. As Weil writes 'It does not rest with the soul to believe in the reality of God if God does not reveal this reality. In trying to do so it either labels something else with the name of God, and that is idolatry, or else its belief in God remains abstract and verbal' (Weil 1977: 133).

Exploring ideas such as these may also have alleviated Edwin's sense of 'time running out', for non-closure renders the finite a relative concept. In short, by coming to recognize himself more comprehensively, to hear the tacit dimension of his life, Edwin may have effected a compassionate transition from notions of 'old order' justice, possibly discovering an order where a man is ultimately accountable, not according to his deeds, but according to his sincerity and self-realization: 'whether he really is what he is to himself, or is to others what he is to himself' (Dunne 1975: 37). Certainly this ideal is commensurate with Edwin's own condemnation of those who 'make theirselves out better than they are.' Avenues thus begin to open whereby the equations of a 'moral economy' may be challenged. Wisdom points to the inadequacies of conventional interpretation. It invites people to a more comprehensive vision of their life's events, allowing them to be seen through 'new eyes' (O'Connell Killen 1997: 13).

This new order, however, does not evade issues of personal responsibility. Since he located his search so firmly within the Judaeo-Christian tradition, Edwin may have found it helpful to consider occasions when Christ subverts conventional justice yet preserves the connection between an act and its perpetrator. Interestingly, these occasions often involve encounters with an 'outsider'. Commenting, for example, on the time a haemorrhaging woman touched Christ's gown (*Mark* Chapter 5, Verses 25–34; *Luke* Chapter 8, Verses 40–1), O'Connell Killen (1997: 13) writes, 'She, the polluted one, touches Jesus, the one the whole crowd recognizes as being anointed with God's power. She takes healing power from the one who, in the conventions of her day, should have been most reviled by the touch of a haemorrhaging woman. But she resists conventions that strip her of her humanity … Faith in this woman is that dual combination of resistance and desire.' Does Edwin not also combine resistance with desire, refusing to accept what the events and circumstances of his life 'ought' to tell him about himself—'I'm not like that person [that is, himself as a murdering soldier] I'd do anything for anyone.' Insofar as it does not allow him to finally make up his mind, to set closure, is his religious uncertainty, not a sign of weakness, but an unrecognized resource?

On another occasion, Christ sidesteps conventional mores by asking a Samaritan woman for a drink (*John* Chapter 4). Her status as stranger amongst other women is established by her fetching the water alone, in the heat of the day. Christ disregards not only the stigma associated with a woman whose partner was not her husband, but contravenes religious and political prohibitions preventing a Jew from speaking to a Samaritan. The descent of the woman's bucket, accompanied by Christ's telling of her life, is a powerful image. The contrapuntal tension of sequential narrative and vertical axis provides not only a symbolic answer to Jung's famous question—'What is your myth, the myth in which you live?' (Jung 1965: 171)—but shows how this 'answer'/water is to be found. It appears that 'there is some profound link … between the story of man's life and the story of his world … to discover his myth he must go deeper into his life than he would were he only going to tell his life story' (Dunne 1975: 50).

Christ presents the woman to herself, not in terms of her 'badness', but in such a way that the sadness of her life is recognized and implicitly accepted as both explanation for and product of her actions. Her failed and inadequate relationships are symbolized by her empty-handed returns to the well. The woman's personal responsibility is undiminished but, perceiving events at a deeper level of understanding, Christ suggests that the link between an action and its ultimate consequences is no longer transparent and predictable. A shift from legalism to compassion fractures the easy symmetry of the 'moral economy'. The woman leaves the well enthused for a new way of living. Urging her neighbours to 'come and see', for language always falls inadequate before reality, she demonstrates that to which Edwin aspires: the knowledge that is not explained but experienced. There is yet a further point to be taken from this story: heart's ease is not, as he supposes, to do with forgetting, but with re-membering (making whole) in a way where it is wiser to judge a man more by what he suffers than by what he does.

Coda

What, in the end, became of Edwin? Did he find peace of heart and mind? Was his dilemma adequately resolved? Did he die 'complete in himself', in that state of being suggested by Carla's bride? Even if unable to declare 'I am', did he real-ize the identity associated with *xenos*, discarding that of the *extraneous* man? Edwin does not provide a 'tidy' illustration of healed ultimate concerns, but neither does he 'disprove' any arguments in favour of his need for spiritual care and support. There was no reconciliation with his children and the rela-tionship with his partner became increasingly strained. His nurses described him as depressed and withdrawn. On the night of his death, when Edie arrived at his bedside she was intoxicated. Taking from her bag a fundamentalist tract, she began to read aloud of 'visions of hell', urging Edwin to 'repent and be saved'. Although nearly unconscious, Edwin was clearly agitated. An emer-gency call was made for the hospice chaplain who, remaining with the couple for some time, gently persuaded Edie to put the tract aside. In the Koran, Allah calls man 'him whom I created lonely' (Picthall 1953: on Sura LXXIV) and it is harder to find a more fitting epitaph for Edwin.

Metaphors of estrangement are powerful mediators of patient experience. Although estrangement may be appreciated as a refuge, it more commonly infers painful personal schisms or difficult feelings of social exclusion. The potential of experiences of estrangement to bear unexpected gifts and insights or to result in unanticipated areas of personal growth, however, ought not to be overlooked. It is the existential implication of any 'gifts' the stranger might bear that points to questions of ultimate meaning and purpose. This is a hori-zon of enquiry that outstrips valuable psychological or sociological percep-tions of human experience and draws attention to a spiritual dimension in much of patients' daily life.

Chapter 13

Recognizing life's 'surplus of meaning'

Introduction

Facet nine is more concerned with the 'unsaid' and the 'unsayable' of this study than the spoken. It acknowledges the right of patients to maintain silence and admits the possibility of interpretative oversights. For example, someone once asked whether Grace—explaining how she charged other children to view her deceased father—might have been speaking obliquely of myself 'peeking' at her experience of dying. Another person immediately spotted in Fig. 9.1 of the sewing woman, a diagonal line extending from the lower left quadrant to the upper right. This effectively divides the work in half so that the woman's head and body are not in the same 'place': a truly liminal predicament which, again, I had not seen. For one attempting to draw attention to aspects of experience that tend to be overlooked, these were sobering contributions. Nevertheless, it was reassuring to learn that notions of liminality could provide at least one other person with a meaningful path through potentially disconnected experiences. Moreover, since this painting occurs in a discussion of metaphors of control, the indivisibility of the prism is again affirmed by the simultaneous illustration of liminality.

Such oversights and 'unsaids' inevitably accompany qualitative research, but the portent of facet nine extends far beyond an injunction for better detective work or the acceptance of some degree of subject privacy or secrecy. Indeed, to understand the 'surplus of meaning' only in these terms reduces any discussion of spirituality, mystery or metaphysical issues to the status of problem solving. The critical issue addressed by facet nine is the collapse of language under the strain of attempting to encapsulate the indefinable. Inarticulacy can intimate matters of some profundity, not a conundrum, and it is hardly surprising that patients prefaced some of their deepest reflections with phrases such as 'this is so hard to put into words …' (Hazel); 'this might sound silly, but …' (Claude); 'I don't know how to say this …' (Mary); or 'this is so difficult to explain …' (Carla). Similarly, professionals not infrequently refer to spiritual care as 'wishy-washy', 'hard to pin down' or 'airy fairy'. The request for a 'tool' to measure spiritual distress frequently arises. In an era character-ized by a craving for order, for permanence, for the 'literal', this is perhaps an expression of discomfort as authentic as that of any patient finding him or herself 'lost for words'. Certainly, the undefined is uncanny and frustrating, but reductionism marks a retreat from vast tracts of human experience. It is the responsibility of any thinking person to demolish attempts to encapsulate that which exceeds the particular and the limited.

We emerge from and return to silence, but the liminality both of human knowledge and human existence is not a 'puzzle' to be solved. It is a mystery with which we must live. Language only captures the surface of life (Ricoeur 1976: 63) and human existence carries degrees of meaning that exceed any interpretation—not as an 'add-on' but as a permeating dimension. The 'stranger' dwells in the heart of the familiar because, at life's deepest moments, something—which is no 'thing'—escapes articulation. A useful analogy exists in the silence that makes music possible, so that, just as Mozart presents tremendous challenges for the master but is generally regarded as 'easy' by the amateur, the deeper one's appreciation of life's unpronounceable aspects, the greater appears their mystery. It is hardly surprising, therefore, if this ninth facet, about which we can say least, is the most pervasive.

Any action, no matter how simple or domestic, carries an ultimate significance as much as it bears physical, social or psychological meaning. Although no demonstrable 'proof' of this has been supplied, it is hoped that the descriptions of patients' sources of meaning, their sense of self, plus the manner in which these have been explored will support the status of 'reliable witness'. The ninth facet thus 'holds' but does not explain why Carla, feeling feverish, described herself as 'spiritually comforted' when her nurse fetched a cool pillowcase. That such a simple gesture should hold such deep meaning, however, supports a major thrust of facet nine: the spiritual does not lend itself to compartmentalization. To be concerned with spirituality, therefore, is not to be concerned with special events but akin to the artist, with the ordi-nary at a depth where conventional interpretations are relativized.

Just as no painting is reducible to its brush strokes or any poem to the sum of its sentences, the prism shares the artist's struggle to achieve the '*ecstatic* moment, the moment of language going beyond itself' (Ricoeur 1978: 249). In this, it demonstrates a fidelity to the experiences of many patients, such as Carla grappling to explain what she meant by the 'really real' or Hazel pointing to her dying flowers as mediators of 'letting go' and personal dissolution. Similarly, Carol and Carla's paintings, Arthur's 'final salute', Debbie's 'inner flame', Tracey's statue and Mary's 'golden door' are not 'puzzles' to be solved but ingenious resorts to the '"perspectival" character of poetic language [which] evokes the excess that surpasses the angle of vision' (Ricoeur 1978: 251). Indeed, by exploiting the creative potential of language and symbol, patients reveal something of the creative potential of life itself (Ricoeur 1978: 254).

This 'creative' abundance permeates every other facet of the prism for there is always something more to be discovered about patient experience. By now, perceptive readers will easily detect the presence of this ninth facet wherever discussions of an ultimate reality have been prompted by patient narrative. Certainly 'perspectival', these discussions have relied upon metaphors of depth, of layers of meaning, of the extraordinary dimension of the mundane, of limit— a horizon of meaning that accommodates and relativizes all others. This relativity, however, ought not to be approached as an exclusively 'quantitative' event, as a means of conceptualizing finite experiences in the light of an infinite backdrop. It also carries 'qualitative' implications insofar as reality acquires a personal significance. Now a radio aerial can be a beacon home and a blue potted plant blazes iridescent in ways never before appreciated. Awareness of an ultimate horizon does not alter life's events but, when perceived before it, their meaning—such as Carol's understanding of her two divorces—may be radically altered.

Metaphors are miniature acts of artistic creation or *poeisis* and this evokes another paradox. All art may mimic or represent life in some way but there is a sense in which good art achieves its effect by operating as 'a memory of what we did not know we knew' (Murdoch 1997: 12). Recollecting his undergraduate naiveté, Bennett (1994: 323) expresses the situation thus: 'poems only tell you what you know already, and I still had it to learn'. Metaphor may have the capacity to name for the first time, but this saying is adventitious. In terms of authenticity, the experience always comes first. This is accommodated both by the language of spirit and the prismatic symbol by their focus on first-order propositions: everything is grounded in the experiences of patients.

Two challenges

Poetic statements have truth without necessarily being 'true' in any removed or free-standing sense. It is, in part, a purpose of this book to rehabilitate this understanding in the realm of palliative care. When patients intimate a 'surplus of meaning' that exceeds conventional physiological, sociological or psychological explanations, they are making a poetic challenge. Meeting this challenge prohibits any foreclosure of existential exploration and requires us to elevate the delimitation of our vision to a status equivalent to our acquisition of more conventional 'facts'. Metaphor and symbol take us to the very limits of our understanding. They belong to what Heaney describes as a 'frontier' where, 'the poem provides a draught of the clear water of transformed understanding and fills the reader with a momentary sense of freedom and wholeness' (Heaney 1996: xv). Currently, however, there exists a generalized attitude of disbelief towards such potential generosity. A suspicious attitude restricts our range of receptivity to the domain of the definitive. In certain fields, such as the trial of new drugs or treatments, this suspicion is entirely appropriate. The metaphors whereby some patients mediate their experience, however, suggest a reality that defies and exceeds this stricture. This augmentation becomes explicit when spiritual awareness is expressed in the religious vocabulary of gift, abundance or presence: 'I believe very strongly in God, very strongly. I've just had too much support over the last fifteen years' (Julia); 'When I prayed, my spirit started burning again. I found it really calming' (Debbie); 'People give me support when they pray for me. I feel uplifted. I know, in some way, that their prayers have helped' (Carla).

The first challenge of facet nine is thus an injunction against any reification of the horizons against which patients' stories are evaluated. In accordance with the aims of the poet, maximum *ecstasis,* not definition, is our ambition. A wry and further challenge is posed by this assumption of the poet's mantle. If poems teach us only what we know already, how do we come to realize that which we unknowingly 'knew' all along? Facet nine does not 'inform' in any conventional sense, but brings us face to face with a paradox raised earlier: we do not see things until they are 'there', but they are only 'there' for us once we see them. Facet nine does not 'answer' this mystery, but serves as a prompt to greater self-awareness and sensitivity towards others, inevitably raising a question whose existential reach requires some contemplation of spiritual or ultimate issues: What kind of a being am I?

Perhaps this is the most challenging gauntlet thrown before readers and some of the means whereby it may be taken up will be considered in the following chapter. Here, it is sufficient to conclude this discussion of the prism's mysterious ninth facet by invoking memories of every other. At the very least, patients' experiences of contingency, liminality, finitude, estrangement, their evocation of archetypal figures and so forth, demand respect and non-denial. Long recorded by disciplines such as psychology or sociology, a closer examination of the prism also divulges that these most human experiences rehearse a 'surplus of meaning' whose theological analysis suggests a spiritual dimension. This may surpass our 'angle of vision' but it ought not simply to be denied. The spiritual thus invites interpretation from all perspectives but prohibits any limitation of enquiry that falls short of the poetic.

Part 4

Implications for spiritual care

Chapter 14

Some inconclusive reflections

Review

Destinations often make greater sense when viewed in the context of their approach and a rear view of this study exposes the pervasive influence of metaphors of conversation. Listening to skilled and experienced practitioners of palliative care initially highlighted how, despite feelings of restraint, the majority seemed to regard conventional empiricism as the only '"legitimate way" of expressing the otherwise "illegitimate" stuff of spirituality in a predominantly materialist, secular, rationalist culture' (Hay and Nye 1998: 129). Human spirituality, however, challenges this cultural dominance and searching for other ways of recognizing patients' spiritual concerns, irrespective of whether they are expressed in religious language, brings one face to face with the artificial boundaries that an exclusive rationality places on human experience. Noticing how patients expressed their thoughts or feelings, observing how their stories could comfort or terrify, witnessing ritualistic behaviour or the symbolic significance of certain artefacts, I became increasingly interested in the ways that 'story making' works, in the sense of providing an understanding of the world, our place in it and pointing towards some mystery or deeper meaning. After listening to only one or two patients, I quickly realized that any understanding of 'story' requires some appreciation of the disclosive potential of metaphor and symbol. I have partly framed this discussion in terms of a comparison of psychological and spiritual discourse, arguing and hopefully later demonstrating that although the former is invaluable, it is the latter that carries one to further depths of meaning. The ultimate authority of the symbol may not lie with the human psyche, but this book also rejects the notion of ultimate foundations grounded in anything essential, representational or definable. This refusal to locate ultimate grounding in the subjectivity of either the individual or the collective deflects any potential accusations of relativism. Although my humanist and experiential methodology shares many features of qualitative sociological research, this attitude of 'non-closure' is a distinguishing feature of theological anthropology. The question of ultimacy has been left open in what, for some, may seem a surprisingly post-modern way. By emphasizing the reasonable, the pragmatic, the negotiated, sometimes the intuited, however, I am not opposed to rational discourse, but regard the empirical as one voice amongst many—not 'the' definitive voice. This is not a move towards the irrational but towards an expanded rationality grounded in those words and deeds of patients that seem to mediate ultimate meaning. With an ethical imperative to listen without distraction and to communicate my impressions as clearly and honestly as possible, metaphors of conversation are thus reasserted. The more patients I encountered, the more I became convinced that the tacit dimensions of their communication were as significant as the more explicit and that paradox should be viewed, not as a problem, but as a valid form of knowing. Otherwise, much of what terminally ill patients experience will continue to be labelled as an 'illegitimate' concern or, in some way, distorted to 'fit' into the ubiquitous rating scale or questionnaire. The confidence underlying this stance is easily traced to contemporary theories of interpretation (Warnke 1987) where metaphors of conversation are again helpful, both encouraging a multi-disciplinary approach and addressing issues of power. One ambition of this book has always been to provide a disadvantaged group with a voice and to draw attention to aspects of their experience that, although spiritually expressive, are often overlooked or discounted. Against those who may belittle a methodology that fails to accurately 'measure' spiritual pain, maintaining that my results will never be considered 'valid', it has been comforting to discover how heavily both the natural sciences and modern physics must rely upon metaphor to refer to that which they cannot define, to name for the first time. This does not mean, however, that my interpretations have been a matter of 'reading' anything 'in' to data. Rather, through its frequent handling, from drawing on diverse academic sources, from conversing with my hospice colleagues and by obtaining suitable therapeutic support for myself—for this data was sometimes deeply moving—I was trying to prepare myself for noticing, in a new way, anything that might proceed from what I was hearing: 'The sense of a text is not behind the text but in front of it. It is not something hidden but disclosed' (Ricoeur 1976: 87).

All of this has led to a position from which I now argue that it is possible to identify at least some of the vocabulary or 'tools' of a non-religious language of spirit. From these 'tools', the metaphors and symbols that mediate patients' experience of terminal illness are created. Although the disclosive potential of these metaphors and symbols extends to a spiritual dimension, definitive statements about this dimension escape their articulation. Nevertheless, I have tried to share my 'hints and guesses' (Eliot 1944: 37) at this excess of meaning by trying to show what I cannot define. To this end, I have resorted to the 'perspectival quality of language' (Ricoeur 1978: 251), of which poetry is the prime exemplar: the language of what one cannot say.

It is this lack of direct access to its object that forces the language of spirit to rely upon symbol and metaphor and gives its moments of clarification and arrival the sense of temporary resting places. Meaning emerges from the inherent tensions of a powerful metaphor with such conviction that its contradictions seem irrelevant. Apprehension of this meaning does not equate with the intellectual mastery of a technical language but with certain unique demands of engagement such as a willingness to tolerate discomfort, a loss of control or an attitude of trust and patience. There is always a quality of the unexpected gift in a novel metaphoric disclosure. Processes of recognition and resonance may be evoked in ways that transcend and expand everyday understanding in unanticipated directions. Metaphor and symbol characterize a language of depth where events become experiences and words operate under a law of diminishing returns. The wiping of a tear, for instance, must be encountered on its own terms. A verbal elaboration is likely to be crudely descriptive or potentially distracting from its deeper meaning. This is a language of the frontier, emerging at the limits of human tolerance and understanding and at dangerous times of transition. The horizons it opens can close as inexplicably as they open, although their memory and experience leave a franca that makes it nigh impossible to return to being exactly as before. The validity of this language of spirit, therefore, is judged less by its content and referent than by its consequences for the individual. It is this entwining with dimensions of personhood that endows the language with its authority, a deeply personal yet seemingly universal and timeless quality.

Considerations of what and how

Hermeneutically speaking, my own 'learning curve' and my research findings are not entirely separable. With my 'divesting methodology' I wanted patients to feel able to take the initiative, to set the pace and ground we should cover. My stance was invitational. After initial courtesies and opening gambits, I usually found little difficulty in encouraging people to talk. I could then follow where they led and many patients expressed relief and gratitude for the opportunity to tell their story in their own way—as distinct from a narrative structured by expectation or necessity. In recounting their experiences of liminality and marginality, of control and letting go or of the mediating influence of the archetypal mother, stranger and so forth, I am reminded of Jasper's observation that although spirituality may speak to us of transcendence, it is firmly rooted in daily life where its glimpse places us in what he calls a 'boundary situation'. He writes 'As existence I am in situations, as possible Existenz in existence I am in boundary situations … the mystic goes on living in the world' (Jasper 1970: 183), continuing 'There is no transcendence without existence … were I to seek pure transcendence without a world, I would lose the boundary situation and sink into an empty transcendence (Jasper 1970: 222). Clearly struggling to find some meaning in their predicament, many of the patients I met were exploring their own 'boundaries', sometimes tackling or trying to avoid profound existential questions: 'What has my life been for?', 'What will happen to me?', 'Why me?', 'Why now?', 'Who am I?' Others made pronouncements worthy of any seer. Judith's observations, for example, draw attention to the human tendency to be distracted from the here and now. They bear a direct comparison with the reflections of the Buddhist master, Thich Nhat Hanh. She remarked 'When we drove to radiotherapy, I'd see someone crossing the road. I would look at them and think, "Do you realize how lucky you are, just to be able to walk?"' As Hanh writes 'Our true home is in the present moment. The miracle is not to walk on water. The miracle is to walk on the green earth in the present moment' (Hanh 1996: 23).

A divesting methodology, however, is not without its dangers. It can evoke the same fears and resistances that lurk whenever one is faced by another's pain, particularly when it seems there is nothing one can 'do' to alleviate the situation. Listening carefully to patients often evoked feelings of personal inadequacy or self-exposure. These are discomforts rooted in the tension that exists between knowing how to behave towards a problem—and knowing what to do about it. 'How' refers to a priority of means and is suggestive of personhood, of the 'innerness' of things, of contemplation. It is a priority exemplified by all non-violent proponents of liberative action, for whom there is no avenue to peace because peace is in every step. Committed primarily to interpersonal values, 'acting, without attachment to the outcome, centred in the stillness of his own being', such a person finds 'end results' a distracting abstraction (MacCuish et al. 1998: 79). 'What', however, is the more traditional, literal and pragmatic prioritization of ends. 'What' expresses a concern for limit and 'getting things done' which, given our innate contingency, is both entirely natural and useful. This delineation, however, risks falling into substantive thinking. 'How' and 'what' are not 'things' opposed, but two dimensions of any approach to a given situation. Contemporary culture nevertheless encourages us to identify totally with our ability to control, to think, to act and the contemplative dimension is submerged. Recalling those patients who experienced feelings of estrangement, of liminality and temporal dislocation, however, it is important to emphasize the relativity of much that we generally assume to be concrete and fixed. This requires a shift in attention towards the personal and Rogers (1975) provides a useful precedence for con-joining this personal dimension with reflective commentary. The retrospective view afforded by this chapter affords a similar opportunity. My own instances of anamnesis or recognition may sound obvious but each was invaluable in the sense of a knowledge experienced, not simply received. In the hope that others may find them useful, I offer the inseparable 'hows' I would have given to myself when embarking upon my methodological 'what'—paradoxically, the route to their discovery.

Firstly, *please allow yourself to experience some confusion.* Constant exposure to death and dying is disorientating and personally challenging. It is impor-tant to be gentle and realistic in one's personal expectations. It also takes time, reflection and sometimes a lot of personal support to develop a certain 'trust' that makes it possible to work in this field, to accept the apparent unfairness of some people's lot. It is reasonable, therefore, to expect to feel challenged at many levels. You will come to see, however, that academic rigour and high professional and ethical standards will foster a critical attitude and an intellec-tual safeguard against sentimentality. Even so, 'if you pray for rain you better get ready for some mud' so that *it would be sensible to regularly meet people with whom you can safely discuss your work.* Find one or two who will be constant intellectual or emotional companions or mentors. If you feel held or secure in this way, the same feelings will be conveyed to those you meet. Consequently, they will find it easier to be forthcoming. Similarly, if you are methodical and confident in executing your professional responsibilities you will exude a sense of security and safety—but take care not to hide behind any 'system' or role, using it to avoid real encounters. Similarly, *when you are listen-ing to others, do not be tempted to appear an expert.* Admit it if you feel out of your depth. Ask for time to think something over. Offer to introduce someone wiser or more experienced than yourself. If people realize that you take them seriously, you will be pleasantly surprised by their response. Nobody will expect you to answer the mysteries of life, but your manner and attitude must make it possible for them to share their story. This will require you to *learn to relinquish your desire to manipulate or control or even to rush in with 'comfort-ing' words* for these responses are more likely to be about self-protection than helping the other. It will be the patient, not you, who decides at what depth to engage in a conversation. Recognizing this will help you to treat them as your equal. If you want to know what they really think or feel, do not ask leading or closed questions. Some people may feel more at ease if they can set the pace, time and place of their meetings with you. Paradoxically, if they feel relaxed about discontinuing their conversation it may make it easier for them to share intimate thoughts and feelings. *Try not to judge a person by anything you may be told.* The radical isolation of personhood prohibits any accurate evaluation of another's 'moral worth'. The point is, you don't know how you would have behaved if you were in their shoes, because you're not the other person. Rather, *it is important to validate the experiences or feelings of the other.* This does not mean reinforcing the actuality of something that cannot possibly have happened or endorsing illegal actions. It means acknowledging, or trying to see, why the person you are listening to might feel, think or behave in a particular manner. Following Murdoch (1997), this is a matter of ethics in practice, of refining one's moral perception by learning to see things from another's point of view.

Pay attention to everything. The 'illogical' line or gesture may speak most deeply. Be very wary, however, of attempting to 'translate' the meaning of a symbolic disclosure. You will not be able to, anyhow, because symbols exceed containment. When people invite you to understand something in the same way a work of art is comprehended, they are not asking for a brutal 'literal' echo or for you to point out what they 'really' mean. They are requesting your companionship in a particular dimension of their reality. Of course, it is acceptable to confirm any specific point, but if someone senses you have tried to 'come alongside' their experiences, as they understand them, they will be satisfied. *But never pretend to understand.* To do otherwise violates the dignity of the other person, as well as your own. It could easily land you in deeper water than simply admitting 'I don't know' or 'I need time to think about that for a while'. Although it can feel dangerous, self-exposure may be the safest, certainly the most honest response you can make.

Please allow yourself to receive thanks and hospitality graciously. This might involve sharing a cup of tea, receiving a smile, sharing a joke or borrowing a book. Of course, it is the simplicity of such actions that makes them so difficult when one feels pressed for time or distracted. There is no need to be afraid of allowing others to see when such actions nourish you. Generosity is not dependent upon physical strength and you will find that the line between giving and receiving is highly permeable. *It is also very important to become comfortable with silence.* If you get into the habit of maintaining even a short period of silence each day you will feel less perturbed when you are invited to share the silence of another. Although this period may initially seem full of distractions, over time, your mind will become more still. Gradually, you will discern that silence has many qualities and functions. Your own story may also come to seem a far more relative affair, so enabling you to become more receptive of the stories of others. Without some experience of silence, its theological interpretation can only seem an abstraction. Even with this experience, there is no guarantee of coming to a theological interpretation.

Be willing to learn new things about yourself. Perhaps you may not like your new personal insights. Perhaps you are less patient, less understanding, more judgemental than you hitherto realized, or maybe you find it hard to accept your good points. Either way, only through some degree of self-knowledge can you learn to be authentic with yourself and others. This is when you will be glad you recruited your supportive 'companions'. Their acceptance will make it easier for you to view yourself realistically and to learn from any shortcomings. Remember, to fire a really strong pot, old or chipped earthenware is ground to dust and mixed with virgin clay. Nevertheless, *do not set yourself unrealistic goals* or become so attached to a particular outcome or direction that you lose sight of the knowledge that unfolds from moment to moment. This knowledge may come from unexpected sources and it is important not to succumb to frustration if 'real life' 'gets in the way' of your plans—because it surely will. Instead, try to be open to learning what it feels like when circumstances say 'no', when you would rather hear 'yes'. This will place you closer to the experiences of patients. You may also find that the painful setback is a vital 'missing piece', a 'moulding interruption' (Nouwen 1998) enabling you to better understand the experience of human finitude. It may re-orientate your attention in some important way.

Try hard not to compare yourself too assiduously against others—carers or researchers. Any reassurance you are seeking will probably be driven by narcissistic tendencies. By deciding to listen deeply, to create the 'space' to meet another person, you will find that you must loosen the ego's stranglehold. This has a liberating quality and effect that makes it possible to learn from others in an easier, freer manner. You must, however, stay 'rooted'. If you can maximize the quality of your presence and attention (really the two are the same) to everyday experiences, you will begin to discover that the 'ordinary' speaks at many levels. Another danger of making comparisons is that the sadness of what you hear may blunt your sympathy for others less *in extremis.*

There will be moments when you feel very aware of the tremendous privilege of sharing time with people who are close to death. Even so, aspects of their care will simply be plain hard work or routine, or about coping with insecurity—your own and other people's. *When you flag, therefore, allow yourself to be nourished by the symbols that you find meaningful.* Finally, *use your common sense*: eat well, exercise, have fun, express your creativity in places other than your work, get your sleep and notice your dreams. Above all, do not lose perspective, because eventually you will realize that you have barely scratched the surface of all there is to learn and understand. You will, however, find that you have been altered by this experience.

In the words of Rogers (1975: 278), 'I think I had better stop here!' The important issue, of course, is whether anything in all this speaks to the experiences of other people. The purpose of this exposition is not to give hard and fast 'rules of approach' (this is anyhow impossible—what 'works' for one will not for another, or even for the same person at another time), but to encourage readers to find the meanings that exist for them in their experience with terminally ill people—to explore their own prioritizations of 'what' and 'how'.

Return to personhood: return to theology

Any call to introspection is a call to personhood and a step towards the existential concerns addressed by theology. Following the philosopher Heidegger's (1962) preoccupations, 'What kind of a being is it whose being consists of caring?' is a question as unavoidable as 'What kind of a being is it whose being consists of understanding?' (Ricoeur 1974: 7). Although primarily committed to the experiences of patients, the following reflections stem from my having witnessed the contingency of much of what we generally take for granted, be it time or identity. The search for somewhere to 'stand' when it seems there is nowhere safe underfoot or for inner confidence and peace when 'things' may ameliorate but they do not reach what ultimately matters, is perhaps one of the greatest challenges facing modern palliative care. This is the situation where, in the words of Hazel, 'You run out of answers—everything falls away. Memory, mind and body, health ... everything ... nothing is left.' In certain cases, the experience of radical limitation, isolation and disengagement occasioned by dying can prompt a yearning for ultimate safety. Such an individual wants to know 'Am I related to anything infinite?' This may be asked openly or emerge as a tacit concern. All experiences of estrangement, for instance, point towards a relevant and challenging paradox. Do 'I' exist both as my thinking, feeling, willing and acting self, but also as 'more-than-this'? Do I realize (to know and to be) a dimension of personhood that is simultaneously myself yet also relativizing Other? Such questions destabilize our customary identification with status or role and, although discomforting, this new insecurity can be symptomatic of a shift towards wholeness, making it possible to think of personhood in terms of symbol, that is, whether finite human creatures mediate anything of an ultimate or infinite significance. This type of speculation, of course, has long been anticipated in story and in her recounting of the *Four rabbinim*, Estes (1992: 32) leads one to wonder whether carers' needs for personal wholeness are not so very different from those of their patients. In the story, four sleeping rabbinim are awoken by an angel who transports them to heaven where they are shown Ezekiel's sacred wheel. On the descent to earth, however, the first rabbi loses his mind, astounded by what he had witnessed. The second rabbi was a cynic, preferring to interpret the event as 'simply a

dream'. The third betrayed the meaning of his experience through its continual analysis. The fourth rabbi, however, was a poet who 'took a paper in hand
and a reed and sat near the window writing song after song praising the
evening dove, his daughter in her cradle, and all the stars in the sky. And he
lived his life better than before.'

Philosophical discussion is rightly prompted by terms such as 'better', but
returning for a moment to the notion of anamnesis, does one not intuitively
recognize what is meant by the change wrought in the fourth rabbi? The story
does not suggest that he is 'trying harder' to be 'good', but that his life is now
more real, more whole, more perfect—in the sense of more complete. Reflecting on the command 'Be ye therefore perfect', Murdoch (1997: 350) suggests
that since the goal of perfection can too easily lead to neurosis, it might be
wiser to say 'Be ye therefore slightly improved', concluding 'It seems to me that
the idea of love necessarily arises in this context. The idea of perfection moves,
and possibly changes us (as artist, worker, agent) because it inspires love in the
part of us that is most worthy.'

Love as the ultimate meaning of the symbolic disclosure (for 'ideas of
perfection' are necessarily expressed in symbolic terms) and living one's life
'better than before' can be approached in terms of faith. This is not faith with
its unfortunate connotations of believing in the unbelievable or of religious
dogmatism. Neither is it faith as an ability, such as being musical, which one
either possesses or not. Faith does not even have to mean a total commitment,
for a total commitment can be its antithesis. Faith owes its derivation to
Hebrew understandings of meaning, of stability and of reliability. The opposite of faith is not unbelief but fear. This owes little or nothing to Plato. Faith is
not about sets of ideas but about ways of being that may involve some element
of surrender. This surrender does not imply any negative self-rejection but
that paradoxical realization of wholeness where 'myself' mediates that which
is also 'more than myself'. Viewed in these terms, faith does not even require a
coherent value system for the meaning and value to which it refers is the
'dimension of the self which unites and integrates. Without it there can be no
wholeness. With it there is a commitment to life and to the enrichment of life
in its highest forms' (Thorne 2001: 87).

There is no suggestion here of approaching the ego as an enemy. A strong
ego, in fact, is necessary to commence and complete certain of life's tasks. Ego
only becomes 'dangerous' if it compromises or distracts from personal wholeness. The professional who is 'driven' by their workload, for example, is easily
distinguished from another who simply has drive and motivation. Finally,
given that we cannot access the spiritual other than through our immediate
circumstances, faith is about being able to 'read' our lives at a deeper level of

meaning. The greater one's 'faith' the further one can 'see'. The fourth rabbi does not experience an isolating perfectionism but is able to relate with others in a more profound way. He still rocks the cradle, he still writes his poetry, but there is a deeper sense of connection. Relieving spiritual distress is thus about helping patients to experience a sense of personal wholeness and interconnectedness where 'the personal' carries a more expansive and inclusive meaning than mere 'individualism'.

Naturally, most of us and for most of the time do not recognize the relativity of our 'ordinary' thinking, feeling and acting selves. When we do, Mayers (1997: 27) describes it as an awakening from 'a deep trance circumscribing awareness, keeping us in a fog about our real identity'. This new perspective carries powerful implications for carers. They may 'want to acquire the "tools of the trade", but real training for service asks for a hard and often painful process of self-emptying. The main problem of service is to be the way, without "being in the way"' (Nouwen 1998: 79). Nouwen is not denouncing personal individuality or promoting negativity, but accepting that carers are vulnerable to fatigue, to making false projections, to finding refuge in inauthenticity—to generally 'getting in the way' if they are submerged in Mayers' 'trance'. Neither is he denigrating professional standards, but recognizing that while the 'tools of the trade' are indispensable, they are insufficient before the total needs of a dying person. Encountering the professional for whom 'good communication' is entirely a matter of acquiring certain skills that give the appearance of being a good listener can be like entering a well-constructed but somewhat inhospitable and empty house. Such communication leaves little space to receive the deepest needs of another. No matter how high standards of care otherwise are, some vital mark is missed. As Hazel commented 'My husband died of heart failure. Now that I'm threatened, I feel strongly that I didn't help him as I might. I was too preoccupied with nourishing soups and all sorts of comforts, but they weren't what he really needed. He wanted communication.'

Randall and Downie (1988: 156) highlight the ethical problems when carers only appear to listen but, as Camilla illustrates, patients are highly discerning: 'I can tell which nurses are really sincere and really feel for you and your loved ones, whereas others ... they don't think of the little things, don't put themselves in my shoes—can't talk, can't move.' The curious bystander at the scene of an accident, or the volunteer whose motivation is that of the voyeur provide helpful analogies. They are easily distinguished from the person who genuinely 'stands by' the injured party—even if there is nothing he can 'do' to help. Even so, despite the reliance of many professional carers upon a vocabulary of 'hopping', 'popping' or 'nipping', or the necessity of asking what is fancied for lunch before the last mouthful of breakfast is swallowed—all of which serve to underline the temporal estrangement of patients, it can take a little while to come 'alongside' another person.

The original impetus for Cicely Saunders' hospice, St. Christopher's, shows how a brief encounter can sustain a lifetime's commitment and that communication may matter more in terms of depth than duration (Clark 2002). Nevertheless, it can still take longer to prepare for than to share a story. Striking the right balance is difficult. Carers may seem to be too withholding, 'some just don't want to get involved in the deep things … maybe they reserve those type of conversations, not for their work, but their private lives' (Julia) or too effusive 'if people are too nice, it's too much to bear' (Camilla). Luke's (1987: 107) reflections on authentic care are invaluable. The carer who reacts to the physical or emotional pain of another with an intense personal emotion will 'either repress what she cannot bear and become hard and unfeeling, or else will increase the sick one's burden through her unconscious identification.' Could this be why Edwin's surgeon broke his diagnosis callously, or why Fred had to lend his crying nurse a handkerchief when he received bad news? By contrast, the one who genuinely cares 'is always deeply concerned; she is compassionate but not invaded by emotional reactions. She is herself changed by the experience through the love that lies beyond emotion. The patient can literally be saved by this kind of "carrying" by another, but can be swamped and pushed deeper into misery by the unconscious reactions of those around her, however well they may be disguised. The difference is subtle but absolutely distinct when experienced' (Luke 1987: 107).

Nearing completion, I see in ways not apparent when 'work was in progress', that despite its inherent Platonism, this notion of a 'love that lies beyond emotion' is a linchpin of this book. It unites life's inexpressible 'surplus of meaning'—the thoughts that are no longer 'thought' for they resist their saying, a theology of personhood—the self that is simultaneously more-than-self and the practicalities of caring for someone who is searching for somewhere to 'stand'. After many conversations with patients, my nascent appreciation of this love and the mystery of its magnetism is perhaps best expressed in Carol's image of eventually finding herself 'sailing on a calm sea'. These reflections, of course, do not qualify as research findings in any orthodox sense, but my model of hermeneutics means they ought not simply to be ignored. It also obliges me to point out that anyone who turns to this book for 'straight answers' about spiritual care will be disappointed for at its heart lie these paradoxes of self and non-self, dissolution and wholeness, reminding me of an elderly Jewish patient who once remarked 'I don't know His name, but I know who He is'. Rather than shy away from silence, confusion, paradox, insecurity and mystery, we need to learn to recognize these as potential heralds of spiritual meaning. To hear clearly, however, we may be required to abandon any expert status, to experience vulnerability, to learn to recognize the illogical as profound or to relinquish the desire to control. This is where understanding becomes a mode of being.

The 'spacious' listener

Silence has the potential to call us to personhood and contemplation can create an 'inner spaciousness' so that an exclusive identification with one's roles and functions does not occur (Nouwen 1998). Although in such territories there are no teachers, only learners, the support of a spiritual guide or counsellor is inestimable for this type of change is not brought about by will power but through a process of 'unselfing'. Nouwen (1998: 3–16) describes the process as a shift from 'suffocating isolation' to a 'receptive' and relativizing solitude where, before one can help another to healing, one must turn to one's self and the place from which such healing comes. For Mary, 'It's when I forget we belong to a wider scheme of things, when I do forget how small we are in comparison with the universe, that's when the fears sneak in.'

There are at least two consequences of realizing one's infinite or relativizing dimension. Firstly, the creation of a 'free and friendly' interpersonal space is fostered where others can be encountered in total acceptance and hospitality. Secondly, increasing personal realization results in and flows from feeling that one is ultimately acceptable—despite all contrary evidence: 'It is the power of being itself that accepts and gives the courage to be' (Tillich 1962: 179). This security makes it possible to affirm others, to reveal to them their own acceptability—no matter what. Spiritual care is not about something abstract. It is about helping another human being to understand that they are lovable. In the words of one patient, 'When you can feel the very life draining from you, what of these existential concerns then? They mean nothing. I want someone to hold my hand.' If the spiritual is a dimension of all experience, it is unsurprising that many patients emphasized the tenderness of small acts performed mindfully—cutting up food discretely, gentleness with the hoist, remembering a limited field of vision, concern for visitors, not rushing. Recalling all that has been said about temporal relativity, no matter how busy a carer may feel, from the dying person's perspective, they have at least the next 10–30 years. It is vital to relax, to sit down with patients, to release the tension that arises from rushing from one task to another and perhaps failing to see what really matters. For carers to have the freedom to behave like this, of course, those who manage and resource services must also value the sometimes less tangible outcomes of care.

When a listener no longer totally identifies with her phenomenal descriptive self, 'she' operates from a space where her relativizing dimension permeates all that she thinks and does. Listening is no longer a matter of technique, but of allowing oneself to be flooded by another's story. Judgemental attitudes are eroded in favour of compassion, for, as Carla's painting of a little dog quivering before a mighty shore (Fig. 7.2) teaches us, we are all on the same beach. Each of us has the same yearning for love and the same capacity to hate. Each of us is capable of the best and the most atrocious of deeds. 'For a compassionate man nothing human is alien, no joy and no sorrow, no way of living and no way of dying' (Nouwen 1977: 41). This does not mean that the listener identifies with the experience of the other. They are not 'hooked' by their story, as in the way one might feel inappropriately culpable after hearing a guilty secret, exposed because regrettable actions of one's own rise to memory in the listening. Neither is there a movement of withdrawal or disinterest. If anything, there is a dissolution of boundary, a dropping of personal defences so that listening takes place in a realm of pure relationship: 'Presence is a reality grounded in some form of communication from one person to another. The community is itself constitutive of the presence, for the communication includes the awareness of two people ... presence is not a static reality' (Cooke 1983: 46).

The temenos was an enclosure though which ancients walked to reach their place of worship. It was a liminal space, neither completely of the 'outside' world, or of the temple. Temenos is an inherently relational concept, helpful for visualizing the characteristic 'space' and heightened sensibility of compassionate listening—the 'time out of time' entered whenever narrative is genuinely shared. In such 'spaces' new and comforting symbols may emerge. Even today, the ablutions of Islam, or crossing with holy water at a church door, mark our intuition of the need to prepare for that which we may not summon, priming us for a potential 'depth encounter'. Thus, it can make sense for a patient to remark 'I'm not strong enough yet to die.'

Once any 'unnecessary' suffering has been resolved, the most precious thing a carer has to offer is the quality of their presence. From the theological perspective, everything about the compassionate listener says 'I am here for you', where 'I' is also 'more-than-myself'. Personal realization of this 'surplus' is an important safeguard against burnout or emotional exhaustion. The carer is not depleted by such encounters, but finds themselves feeling nourished. They discover that although there is a 'deep aloneness that human companionship cannot seem to take away ... [it can], nevertheless be given and received. And when it is given and received, he finds that it becomes an all-oneness, a wholeness. To receive his wholeness from another he finds that he must listen to the whole other, not only to what is said but to what is unsaid and perhaps cannot be said. At the same time, giving heed to what is said and unsaid as well as to what is said, he gives a wholeness to the other' (Dunne 1983: 115). Patients do not only receive and carers do not only give. It is often wiser not to probe another's deep and personal needs too curiously, but rather to simply trust that listening, kindness and gentleness will be experienced as what is required—will reach the hidden place. We all feel good about ourselves after spending time with a friend. They do not need to tell me that I am great, or to attempt any kind of analysis. Simply from being in their company, I feel affirmed. Health care professionals are not patients' friends, of course, but it is possible to experience—if not always to create—this kind of reciprocity.

I once sat with an elderly man at the bedside of his unconscious wife. Taking from his wallet some photographs of her as a young girl in summer shorts, as a radiant bride and then as a sophisticated woman, he confided 'this feels all wrong, it's taking so long, now I'm just waiting for her to die, there's nothing I can do.' Tears came to his eyes when I suggested that perhaps he was finding it so difficult because he was not only waiting 'for' his wife but 'with' her. I wondered whether, even unconscious, she might sense his presence as gift, as a vigil that no one but himself could make. This simple reframing seemed meaningful, particularly the dignity of the word 'vigil', which he repeated. Squeezing my hand for a moment, he replied 'Yes, I can always know, at least I did this.' As for myself, I felt strangely comforted and deeply moved by his touch.

Experiences like this, or the washing of Claire's hands, may not be ossified: 'preserved until required'. This level of understanding has to happen in order for it to be. It is entirely gratuitous and not of our own making—although we may prepare. Thus, in our most significant interactions, the primacy and generosity of love is affirmed. Nevertheless, recalling that it requires at least a lifetime to learn how to be 'the way that care is given without getting in the way' (Nouwen 1998: 79), even situations as tragic as that of Edwin's do not necessarily contradict the changelessness of love, but imply a certain opacity, an inability to see the 'end' of his story: 'If the doors of perception were cleansed, Everything would appear ... as it is, infinite' (Blake 1972: 154).

In a culture that is geared to ends, often before means, it can be hard to accept that spiritual care is about 'preparing for an experience we cannot evoke' (Louth 1994: 3). Much as Edwin was not required to create his own religious belief, to guard against exhaustion, despair and unrealistic expectations it is important for carers to recognize the limits of their own responsibility for patients' well-being. Even if we can accept that the 'time' of Edwin's story may not be 'our time', that its final apotheosis may not be our business, realizing one's personhood in ways that inform high professional standards is still a tall order. There is a sense in which I may not accompany another through territories that I have not, to some extent, explored myself. I must be able to contemplate my own mixed feelings about death, be willing to enter uncomfortable and perhaps unfamiliar territories. Otherwise, when listening to patients who express their thoughts and fears, I will be like the character Nasrudin in an old Sufic tale. Nasrudin sees a man searching the ground beneath a street lamp and asks if he has lost something. 'Yes, my key,' comes the reply. 'And you think you dropped it here?' 'Oh no, over there—but there's light here.' It takes time to become accustomed to the dark and it helps if carers have a personal knowledge that it is possible for spiritual distress to lead to liberation and growth. Without trivializing the anguish of patients, this is expressed in an attitude of calm and an essential trust in the order of life, a belief that somehow, 'all will be well'. Even if they cannot share the 'all will be well' world view, their preparedness to share pain will bring comfort and perhaps enhance their patients' spiritual awareness. Certainly, for both patients and their 'families', without needing to 'do' anything special, a calm carer is a powerful and comforting testimony to the naturalness of dying. This attitude is born of a familiarity with the issues that arise when someone is dying and the ability to be in an area characterized by uncertainty and searching. Although it is hard to apply 'labels' to such people, this type of presence is surely best exercised by those whose personhood or mode of being, like that of the fourth rabbi, is most realized or conscious. It is hard to see how I can accompany anyone facing deep questions of meaning and identity without some prior contemplation of my own personhood. In order to offer hospitality it helps to have once been a stranger (Nouwen 1998: 45) and, in a famous anticipation of contemporary psychology, 'I may not love unless first I know myself as loved' (St Teresa of Avila). Insights such as these stem from a response at the level of one's total being. They are less about academic mastery than a new engagement with life, about developing a receptivity and transparency not dissimilar from that of the fourth rabbi. Furthermore, although to understand anything is to be changed, these reflections are primarily a gesture of hospitality. If an empty house is unwelcoming, they are how I have come to 'inhabit' this work. The various 'showings' of patients have led me to a point where I can assert that to be human is to live symbolically. In varying intensities of presence we each mediate an ultimate dimension of personhood; we are all 'worth' more than our worst action. This in no way diminishes the uniqueness of each individual but, since the origin of this dimension lies beyond human genesis, to be finite is also to be gift. When the stranglehold of identification with one's phenomenal acting self is loosened one realizes that, to some degree, relationships with other people are also constituted by this ultimate dimension—where all participants are received at every moment. This acceptance better enables one to affirm and to accept others. Finally—notwithstanding its inevitable distortions, occlusions and perversions—each of these insights is underwritten by glimpsing the primacy of love in all areas of human experience. It is possible to argue for 'an historical and eschatological order where love is prior to knowledge' (Davis 1994: 12), Murdoch can comment on 'that part of us which is most worthy' and many patients under the mantle of seer make pronouncements such as Gregory's: 'happiness will flow after being kind and being thoughtful. If we were surrounded by kind and thoughtful people what a lovely world this would be. This is my biggest lesson in all this.'

Aspects of the above, of course, read as an abstract presentation of much religious thought: Eckhart on the 'divine spark within', Hebraic notions of 'devekut'— the idea of God as ground of our being and to whom we cleave; understandings of universal Buddha nature. For some, this perhaps gives rise to wondering whether it is possible for an atheist to meet spiritual needs. Such a question, however, betrays the moralist and rationalist tendencies of much Western thought. It reflects a sense of qualification: 'you have to be this, before you can do that', and expresses a naïve urge to tidy the complexities of human experience. If there is any real cause for concern, it must surely be the attitude of closure to which both religious people and atheists can be equally vulnerable. Either camp can prompt the wariness that any fundamentalist expression arouses. Agnosia, the attitude of simply not knowing may be less suffocating or threatening for a patient who is anyhow more likely to be searching for companionship than for an 'expert'. In the quest for ultimate meaning, however, even the wise are relative beginners and Jainism or Buddhism remind us that not all spiritual paths speak in (mono)theistic terms. Anyhow, as the patients in this study demonstrate, 'God talk' is of the second order. Experience comes first. It is possible to mediate spiritual values without needing to make their source explicit. If my conversations with patients have taught me anything, it is the inherent ambiguity of human experience. Spiritual or human concerns come down to 'yes/true' or 'no/false' statements only with great difficulty and most patients seem to recognize this. Acknowledging the impossibility of imposing any closure on such concerns leaves space for a creative future response, even though it may lie beyond our ken. Those who wish to respond with sensitivity to the total needs of the dying person are not called upon to resolve doctrinal issues or to make dogmatic statements, but to realize their own wholeness as far and as authentically as they are able. The admonition received by the first Catholic nun to become a Zen master seems relevant. Sister Elaine and her Roshi's (teacher's) wife were chatting. The latter likened her friend to Bodhidharma, the first Zen teacher in the Philippines. Recalling his 9 years of sitting alone, Sister Elaine responded

"'I wonder how long it will be before Eka [the first disciple] comes". At this, the Roshi drew himself up to his full stature and looked at me gravely. "I don't think your concern is about Eka, but whether or not Bodhidharma will be there!'" (MacInnes 1996: 37).

'Attention': a potential vehicle for spiritual care

Insofar as this book tries to reflect on the inexpressible, it is a treatise in absurdity. Introducing 'attention' as emblematic of spiritual care will, I hope, reassure any readers for whom the absurd is, by now, becoming just a little too absurd. My brief has been to identify a language of spirit and what terminally ill people use it to say, not to write a compendium of 'spiritual tactics'. My inability to see beyond any 'furthest horizon' also absolves me from providing any universal theory of spiritual care. Nevertheless, to say nothing about meeting patients' spiritual needs would be to fail my own communicative injunction. Here, 'attention' is my chosen avenue for approaching the practicalities of welcoming, comforting and learning from others. Carrying implications of giving heed, of attending, of consideration, of thought and observant care, plus an erect attitude of readiness, 'attention' is a concept that 'pulls' in two directions. It simultaneously implies the exclusive narrow focus typical of intense concentration with a widening and inclusive sensibility advanced by theological or spiritual interpretations of personhood and communication. Spiritual teachers of all ages emphasize the 'receptive' quality of a calm and serene attitude developed in tandem with 'active' qualities of deliberate effort and conscious awareness. 'Attention' thus satisfies those bewildered by the popularity of quasi-mystical notions, such as Buber's (1958) *I and Thou*—people who want to concentrate on the 'here and now' and 'nothing airy fairy', while others are reassured by the unity of 'self'/'more-than self' reported by practitioners of inner attentiveness, meditation or prayer. It would be a mistake, however, to regard these two understandings of attention as oppositional. Most traditions speak of individuals who become fully realized, not by following complex procedures, but through living in a state of utter simplicity and fully present to the near at hand. In Christian terms this means becoming as a little child, or in Zen, when you carry water, carry water. If a boomerang never really 'leaves' because it always returns to the point of its ejection, no matter how far 'attention' enters theological 'air space', it does not threaten 'common sense' for it is a concept belonging both to dimensions of 'what' and 'how'.

Borrowing from Simone Weil, Murdoch (1997: 327) points to feminine implications of waiting, of watching, of things coming to fruition in secret, of a penetrative but non-analytical 'just and loving gaze'. Most sensitive carers can appreciate such qualities—even if they baulk at the notion of attention as 'a skill we can develop and a gift we can receive that unifies the Absolute and everyday life' (Mayers 1997: 62). Whether care assistant or surgeon, it makes sense that one's response to a given situation is almost certainly partially predetermined by the quality of one's attention. The idea that this usually involves some degree of 'self-forgetting' is also highly accessible. Rather like the women in Figs 9.1 and 9.2, who has not 'lost' themselves when deeply engrossed in some task, simultaneously oblivious of time's passing? Furthermore, most people understand that 'Looking at other people is different from looking at trees or works of art ... a loving look cherishes and adds substance, a contemptuous gaze withers' (Murdoch 1997: 463). Attention thus summons us to ethics. It is an 'instrument of moral perception' (Murdoch 1997: 463) because 'different interpretations of our human experiences produce different understandings of "the human" and different understandings of this meaning cause the very reality of being human to be different' (Cooke 1983: 36). Two people may thus meet the same frail and elderly man but where one welcomes the wisdom of experience, the other feels repulsed or irritated. Almost certainly, sooner or later, the man will detect the difference in attitudes. This affects his experience of himself and the value he places on his own life. The very reality of his being human has been caused to be different. Acts of care are not just the avowal and expression of a commitment to attend to another, but powerful statements of moral value, an ethical confirmation of worth and potential, regardless of physical condition.

Not every dimension of a person's life is immediately available to exterior appearances. Some can only be seen by the eye of love. Love is not employed here in any sentimental sense, as a matter of simple attraction or transient emotion, but as an expression of committed attention. Committed attention enables carers to recognize in patients' words and deeds even the most tentative indications of their spiritual concerns, much as the loving adult understands that the child handling a stone is 'really' playing with a car. There is an ancient idea that the eye of the mind sees concepts, the eye of the body sees objects, but the eye of the heart sees by entering, by participating in the situation of another on their own terms. Attention thus becomes that quality of presence that says 'I am here for you', revealing to the other that they are lovable. This recognition carries a tremendous potential and, as carers, 'it is our role to help people to make connections in their lives (not to make connections for them): to make connections between their human experiences and the deep longings of their spirit, to make connections between their relationships with others and their struggles within, to make connections which lead to the integration of the psychological, emotional and spiritual dimensions of the self. This is best accomplished through listening' (McNamara 1983: 73). People need to ask their own questions, to water their own seeds, not to feel bombarded by someone else's answers. Otherwise, as one young woman who attended St Christopher's day centre wrote, 'their meaning will merely float about in front of your eyes. Your dictionary will not help you.'

The attentive carer is not only a first-rate professional and possibly a 'spacious listener', they are skilled in creating comfortable physical surroundings and a culturally hospitable milieu. They may not be called upon to perform anything particularly complex but as patients constantly reiterate, 'committed attention' from one who is able to 'see' deeply makes all the difference: 'If I get the pain and ask for a tablet, they give me one. Privacy is a great help. Here, I can talk, and I need to. I need time to accept what's going to happen. At the same time, I need encouragement not to give up. All this takes the anxiety away, and knowing I can come back if I need to is a great help' (Edwin). Performed attentively, the simplest action has a potential to hold life's fracturing experiences, to place them against a wider horizon that, even briefly, can be deeply healing. Nevertheless, there still remains an element of gift in meeting another at their deepest level of meaning. Adequate pain relief (whose development has resulted from the scrutinizing attentions of clinical research), a hospitable environment, familiar food and approachable people, however, are all expressions of 'making space' for another. Combined, these make for an atmosphere of trust and acceptance, all of which may predispose towards inner discoveries of meaning and personhood.

Prompts, questions, and possible developments

Given that palliative care frequently takes place in diverse and often complex circumstances, thinking in terms of prompts and questions is often more helpful than approaching situations with ready-made answers. Faced with someone who is dying, carers need to wonder: 'In what or whom does this person trust?', 'How can we give him control or help his need for accountability?', 'Does this person demonstrate or express a desire for some form of reconciliation?', 'How does she communicate her feelings?', 'How can we nurture her capacity to give and to create?', 'Is he anxious about friends or family, perhaps even a pet?', 'How does she seem to be making sense of what is happening?'. This Socratic approach is intended to foster attention, not only towards others but, equally importantly, towards oneself: 'Am I the kind of person I would like to have near me when I am dying?', 'How do I recognize my own needs?',

'Do I have a sense of my own spirituality?', 'Do I ever contemplate my own death?', 'If I do, how do I feel?', 'How do I cope with the 'lost' opportunity?', 'Where do I find support?', 'How do I stay alongside the anguish of individuals and families?', 'Am I taking power away, diminishing this person's coping ability?', 'What are my motives for this work?', 'Am I avoiding any 'little deaths' in my own life by choosing to work with people who are terminally ill?'. This is not a quest for speculative theory but a movement towards an embodiment of good practice in ways that stem from and contribute to personal growth. Self-reflection is sometimes painful and it is interesting to observe one's physical response to such questions—whether one becomes tense, nervous, decides to break for a coffee, yawns or simply feels distracted. Committed attention may be akin to love but when it is directed towards oneself, it sometimes may feel as though it dismembers before it makes whole. It was not for nothing that St John requested the journeying Dante to show, 'how many are the teeth whereby this love of thine does bite' (Luke 1989: 180). Close personal examination can result in feelings of confusion. It may seem as though one's familiar self is being 'broken up'. As one's self-awareness enlarges there is a sense in which this is true. Personal distress may signal caution but it can also indicate an awakening and movement towards wholeness, greater personal realization and ultimate well-being. Certainly, if one wishes to help another to wholeness it is essential to be aware of one's own 'fragmenting tendencies'. Equally, it is important not to berate or judge oneself harshly. Simply becoming aware of the quality of one's touch, one's presence or even of how one breathes can be sufficient to foster positive changes both towards oneself and others without any further need to 'do' anything elaborate. Of course, support is vital during intense periods of personal growth and in some instances it is wise to recruit the help of an experienced and discerning counsellor or spiritual director.

The artistic impulse is universal and no environment can be truly hospitable if it fails to recognize that human beings need beauty to thrive. Where palliative care takes place in an institutional setting, culturally accessible works of art may help to place present troubles in less distressing perspectives. Good art will inspire and comfort. Similarly, natural symbols—plants, water, stones or silent spots where people may simply be—should be accessible to carers and patients alike. Sensitive design and décor mitigate against the effects of physical limitation and help to prevent cultural differences from rendering people strangers where they should feel at home. Organizational attention, however, only begins with the physical environment. Ways of fostering interdisciplinary honesty so that people can safely exchange thoughts and feelings must be addressed. The attentive organization needs to ask 'How are staff supported in the long term and in the event of a crisis?', 'How is personal/professional development facilitated?', 'How does this organization support those who find they are unsuited to palliative care yet harbour confused feelings about leaving?' An attentive organization will embody a positive commitment to principles of equal opportunity and anti-discrimination, both in terms of employment practice and care provision. All groups should feel welcomed, respected and free to express their identity and be encouraged to pass both negative or positive comments in the conviction that they will be heard and acted upon. Organizational support also means 'ring-fencing' time and physical locations for investment in deepening attention. Resources that address the breadth of human experience should be to hand: relevant audiotapes, literature from all genres, educational videos, appropriate 'general release' films. Structured courses that flag up spiritual needs as a concern for all staff should be regularly programmed. Assuming a suitable level of confidentiality and support, it is essential that experiential exercises, self-reflection and discussion are core features of any focus on spiritual care. Individual professions have specific needs, but mixing different groups and grades can foster unity and, perhaps for some, a realization that wisdom does not always come with a certificate. Suitable follow-up is vital, for the development encouraged by such courses is not like learning 'facts'. Deep insights can have birthing pains and take some time to crystallize. Again, this process requires support and encouragement from someone familiar with such processes who understands what it means to attend deeply to the learning of another. In such an area, the good 'teacher' must personify much of their 'material'.

It is impossible to produce definitive statements on spiritual issues but if care is to be sensitive and appropriate, carers need to respect whatever elicits a sense of awe or holiness for a patient. Death must be allowed to occur in a culturally sensitive manner, letting those close to patients do whatever they feel is helpful. This requires a very personalized approach, openness and flexibility on the part of professionals and a willingness to respond to the criticisms and suggestions of particular groups that claim to represent patient or family interests. Unless both organization and individual carers embody these attitudes, it is unlikely that all patients, especially those from minority backgrounds, will be able to say 'Here I am—and it's alright'. Interestingly, in several religious traditions 'Here I am' has the sense of 'I'm ready—call me', as in Isaiah's reply to the call to prophesy. In this context, therefore, it is particularly important to recognize 'home' as being an experience of comfort and of readiness. To arrive at such a position may require an individual to engage in an inner process, a focusing and reflection on the events, non-events, regrets or missed opportunities of their life. This is a sifting akin to processes of story telling and the official curriculum vitae may diverge from the private inner narrative. A strong sense of personal accountability may precipitate feelings of failure or of besmirched personal integrity. It is important for professionals to respond sensitively when patients raise apparently 'silly' questions for these may mask painful events or memories. Even if personal reconciliation between family members or friends is impossible, there may be some move towards self-forgiveness and self-acceptance. Those who have failed to forge loving relationships in life may find consolation in the knowledge that it is enough to die with the desire for good, that the potential for this desire is a positive that ought not to be excluded from any process of self-evaluation.

While it is recognized that some symbols carry universal or archetypal meanings, they should never to be imposed on patients but must emerge in the context of a caring relationship where they can safely explore what matters most to them. Such a relationship is founded on an attitude of trust: professionals who are able to trust in their colleagues and their own ability to swim in a tide of uncertainty and patients who feel that those who care for them are trustworthy. Where care is provided in an institutional setting, such trust is fostered not only in the individual consultation but also by the attitudes and manner of all staff, the accessibility and pleasantness of the environment and in all manifestations of the prevailing ethos.

The spiritual may be a dimension of all human relationships, but on a palliative care team it is important for someone to be specifically responsible and accountable for spiritual care. Confidential individual support for both staff and patients from someone—and here I stick my neck on the line—trained in pastoral theology should be available. 'Pastoral', because this implies a 'cultural' credibility, a prior relevant experience or 'ticket of entry' from another field— perhaps nursing, medicine, social work. 'Theology', partly because it combines a wide and unbounded literature: philosophy; ethics; psychology, the social sciences and various schools of counselling; and art and sacred texts from all traditions, with an understanding of both formal and informal symbol systems, ritual, prayer and meditation. Local situations may vary, but this role is traditionally associated with an ordained chaplain, usually Anglican. Given the complexities of post-modern society, however, perhaps it is time to develop a greater openness to contemporary human experience and for a less historically conditioned look at spiritual care. Diversity is not a threat to spiritual care but presents many valuable opportunities. As Davis (1994: 122) writes 'pluralism is not correctly understood as a consequence of relativist and secularist principles but as a mode of experiencing transcendence. Pluralism is the tribute that finitude owes to the infinite.' Returning briefly to metaphors of conversation, the patterning of spiritual care should be informed by many voices.

More important perhaps than any status as an unsentimental and analytical thinker, an authentic pastoral theologian should be willing to experience a powerlessness and relativity far removed from professional mystique. In terms of their own 'unselfing' or spiritual development, they must 'walk their talk'. Critically, if they walk it well they will rarely need to 'speak' as they help both carers and patients to make their own connections. Other dimensions of this role require contribution to education programmes and ethical debate and the forging of links with the representatives of various faith groups in the local community. Such a person has the potential to offer 'distinct benefits to the four components of any healthcare system: the patients and their family members, the professional healthcare staff, the organization itself and the community within which it resides' (VandeCreek and Burton 2001). Clearly, issues of accountability, spheres of competence, resource allocation and outcome measurement cannot simply be ignored and although imaginative ideas are beginning to emerge (Cobb 2001), their detailed examination exceeds these parameters. The main point I wish to make is that unless transparency to an ultimate horizon is valued in principle by employers, there is a danger that providers of palliative care will come to regard spiritual issues as a purely subsidiary interest of psychotherapeutic support, an impoverishment this book strongly resists.

Nevertheless, there is still much room for investment, research and pedagogic development around the spiritual needs of terminally ill people. As Cobb suggests, a multi-disciplinary body representing relevant aspects of academia, the social sciences, philosophy, psychology and theology, various religious representatives and those involved in actual patient care could provide a forum for further discussion and perhaps bring valuable local initiatives to wider attention. Eventually, such a body might even lead to recognized standards for the accreditation and ongoing support and development of spiritual or pastoral care workers. Useful lessons could perhaps be learned from the USA where spiritual care has been a cross-curricular concern for longer. In the multi-cultural UK, work on different cultural expressions of spiritual need is an imperative. Given that most people find their deepest personal meaning in relationships, understanding 'family' dynamics is also an essential requirement of spiritual care. Since their tenacity frequently causes distress, research into ways in which 'families' might be helped to 'let go' and what this would mean for all parties, seems overdue. It would also be interesting to see if the language of spirit described here is recognizable in other contexts or at an earlier stage of the terminal patients' 'career'. As professional carers, for instance, how do we express our spirituality? What are the implications of this for patients and for each other? Many of the topics raised by this study—silence, temporality, estrangement—are sufficiently challenging to occupy their own texts and it would be interesting to see some further development of these themes.

These suggestions may 'barely scratch the surface', but suggestions cut adrift from specific circumstances express an emancipatory zeal I am keen to side step. At its close, this book finds itself not on bedrock, but at further frontiers. This is perhaps the most profitable, honest and exciting place for it to be, given the artificiality of any 'conclusions' where spirituality is concerned. Universalism may be the currency of rationalism but mine is a 'reasonable' phenomenology and I am satisfied with generalizations: spiritual care is about a broadening of existential horizons, a finding of support when it would initially appear there is none and a relationality between carer and cared-for that is similar to the 'strange and beneficent process in marriage by which a couple can, in the words of A. D. Hope, the Australian poet, "move closer and closer apart"' (Bayley 1998: 39). I have tried to support these generalizations by pointing to a 'language of spirit' and showing how it can both mediate and express ultimately significant disclosures. Thankfully, receptivity towards the disclosive potential of metaphor and symbol seems to be increasing in palliative literature (Gillon 1997; Scott 1997; Roy 1999), even the need to define seems to be losing ground where existential issues are concerned (Boyd 2000; Byrne 1999; McGrath 1999). After participating in study days and courses for palliative care workers, I also know that the general thrust of much that has been written here evokes recognition and relief when people find their own (previously 'illegitimate') suspicions of meaning validated. This anamnesis honours every patient who so generously contributed to this book. These patients voice an opportunity to make a positive difference to the care of other terminally ill people. They show that it is possible to recognize spiritual needs, growth, and awareness even when they are not expressed in religious language. Gratitude seems an appropriate note on which to end.

References

Ainsworth-Smith, I. and P. Speck (1982). *Letting go: caring for the dying and bereaved.* SPCK, London.

Albery, N. (ed.) (1997). *Poem for the day.* Sinclair-Stevenson, London.

Astrov, M. (1962). *American prose and poetry.* Capricorn Books, New York.

Bach, S. (1990). *Life paints its own span: on the significance of spontaneous pictures by severely ill children.* Daimon Verlag, Einsiedeln.

Bailey, R. (1987). *Thomas Merton on mysticism.* Image Books. Doubleday and Co., New York.

Balarajan, R. (1995). Ethnicity and variation in the nation's health. *Health Trends* 27: 114–19.

Barby, T. and P. Leigh (1995). Palliative care in motor neurone disease. *International Journal of Palliative Care Nursing* 1: 183–8.

Baruch, G. (1981). Moral tales: patients' stories of encounters with the health profession. *Sociology of Health and Illness* 3: 275–96.

Bayley, J. (1998). *Iris: a memoir of Iris Murdoch.* Duckworth, London.

Beckett, W. (1995). *Meditations on silence.* Dorling Kindersley, London.

Bennett, A. (1994). *Writing home.* Faser and Faber, London.

Berger, P. L. (1969). *A rumour of angels—modern society and the rediscovery of the supernatural.* Double Day and Company, New York.

Berger, P. L. (1997). *Redeeming laughter: the comic dimension of human experience.* Walter de Gruyter, New York.

Bettelheim, B. (1991). *The uses of enchantment. The meaning and importance of fairytales.* Penguin Books, London.

Bharati, A. (1985). The self in Hindu thought and action. In *Culture and self: Asian and Western perspectives* (ed. A. J. Marsela, G. de Vos and F. Hsu), pp.185–230. Tavistock Publications, New York.

Bielenberg, C. (1984). *The past is myself,* Transworld.

Blake, W. (1972). The marriage of heaven and hell. In *Blake: complete writings.* Oxford University Press.

Bolen, J. S. (1996). *Close to the bone. Life threatening illness and the search for meaning.* Scribner, New York.

Boulad, H. (1991). *All is grace. God and the mystery of time.* Crossroads Publishing Company, New York.

Boyd, K. J. (1993). Short terminal admissions to hospice. *Palliative Medicine* 7: 289–94.

Boyd, K. M. (2000). Disease, illness, sickness, health, healing and wholeness: exploring some elusive concepts. *Journal of Medical Ethics: Medical Humanities* 26: 9–17.

Bronfen, E. (1992). *Death, femininity and the aesthetic.* Manchester University Press.

Brown, J. and A. Williams (1993). Spirituality and nursing: a review of the literature. *Journal of Advances in Health Care* 4: 42–66.

Brun, B., E. W. Pederson *et al.* (1993). *Symbols of the soul. Therapy and guidance through fairy tales.* Jessica Kingsley Publishers, London.

Buber, M. (1947). *Between man and man.* Beacon Press, Boston.

Buber, M. (1958). *I and Thou.* T. and T. Clark, Edinburgh.

Byrne, M. (1999). A humbler approach to the unknowable? *Progress in Palliative Care* (7)1: editorial.

Callanan, M. and P. Kelley (1992). *Final gifts: understanding and helping the dying.* Hodder and Stoughton, London.

Camus, A. (1981). *L'Etranger [The Outsider],* Hamish Hamilton.

Cassell, E. J. (1982). The nature of suffering and the goals of medicine. *New England Journal of Medicine* 306: 639–45.

Charmaz, K. (1983). Loss of self: a fundamental form of suffering in the chronically ill. *Sociology of Health and Illness* 5: 168–95.

Charmaz, K. (1991). *Good days, bad days: the self in chronic illness and time.* Rutgers University Press, New Jersey.

Chopra, D. (1997). *The path to love.* Rider Books, London.

Clark, D. (2002). *Cicely Saunders. Founder of the hospice movement. Selected letters 1959–1999.* Oxford University Press.

Clark, S. H. (1990). *Paul Ricoeur.* Routledge, London.

Cobb, M. (2001). *The dying soul. Spiritual care at the end of life.* Open University Press, Buckingham.

Connell, C. (1988). *Something understood— art therapy in cancer care.* Wrexham Publications, London.

Connell, C. (1992). Art therapy as part of a palliative care programme. *Palliative Medicine* 6: 18–25.

Cooke, N. (1983). *Sacraments and sacramentality.* Mystic, Connecticut.

Cowan, R. J. (1991). The spiritual dimension of patient care: obligation, necessity or optional extra? Unpublished dissertation for B.Sc. (Hons) in Nursing Studies. King's College, University of London.

Cowman, S. (1993). Triangulation as a means of reconciliation in nursing research. *Journal of Advanced Nursing* 18: 788–92.

Cox, M. and A. Theilgaard (1987). *Mutative metaphors in psychotherapy: the aeolian mode.* Tavistock Publications, London.

Crossan, J. D. (1975). *The dark interval. Towards a theology of story.* Argos Publications, USA.

Cutcliffe, J. R. (1995). How do nurses inspire and instil hope in terminally ill HIVpatients? *Journal of Advanced Nursing* 22: 888–95.

Dahlke, R. (1992). *Mandalas of the world: a meditating and painting guide.* Sterling Publishing Company, New York.

Dalley, T. (1989). *Art as therapy. An introduction to the use of art as a therapeutictechnique.* Tavistock/Routledge, London, New York.

Dass, R. and P. Gorman (1985). *How can I help?* Rider, London.

Davidhizar, R. and J. Newman Giger (1994). When your patient is silent. *Journal of Advanced Nursing* 20: 703–7.

Davis, C. (1994). Religion and the making of society: Essays in social theology. Cambridge University Press.

de Caussade, J. P. (1981) *The sacrament of the present moment*. Fount Publications, London.

de Hennezel, M. (1997). *Intimate death: how the dying teach us to live*. Little Brown and Company, London.

Dillistone, F. W. (1955). *Christianity and symbolism*. Collins, London.

Donaldson, M. (1992). *Human minds: an exploration*, Penguin, London.

Douglas, M. (1978). *Purity and danger. An analysis of concepts of pollution and taboo*. Routledge and Kegan Paul, London.

Dreyfus, H. L (1991). *Being-in-the-world: a commentary on Heidegger's being and time. Division I*. MIT Press. Cambridge, Massachusetts.

Dunne, J. S. (1975). *A search for God in time and memory*. Sheldon Press, Southampton.

Dunne, J .S. (1983). Time and myth. A meditation on storytelling as an exploration of life and death. University of Notre Dame Press, London.

Dyson J., M. Cobb *et al.* (1997). The meaning of spirituality: a literature review. *Journal of Advanced Nursing* 26: 1183–8.

Edinger, E. F. (1973). Ego and archetype. Individuation and the religious function of the psyche. Penguin Books, New York.

Eichelman, B. (1985). Hypnotic change in combat dreams of two veterans with post traumatic stress disorder. *American Journal of Psychotherapy* 142: 112–14.

Eliade, M. (1957). *Myths dreams and mysteries*. Harvill Press, London.

Eliade, M. (1979). *Patterns in comparative religion*. Sheed and Ward, London.

Eliot, T. S. (1933). *The use of poetry and the use of criticism: studies in the relation of criticism to poetry and England*. Faber and Faber, London.

Eliot, T. S. (1944). *Four quartets: Burnt Norton, East Coker, The Dry Salvages, Little Gidding*. Faber and Faber, London.

Ersek, M. (1992). Examining the process and dilemmas of reality negotiation. *IMAGE Journal of Nursing Research* 24: 19–22.

Estes, C. P. (1992). Women who run with the wolves. Contacting the power of the wild woman. Rider Books, London.

Faber, H. (1971). *Pastoral care in the modern hospital*. SCM Press, London.

Fairbairn, W. R. D. (1954). *An object relations theory of the personality*. Basic Books, New York.

Family resources survey for Great Britain (1995–95). Chapter 6: Carers. Department of Social Security. HMSO, London.

Fawcett, T. (1970). *The symbolic language of religion*. SCM Press, London.

Field, D., J. Hockey *et al.* (1997). *Death gender and ethnicity*. Routledge, London.

Fine, M. (1994). Working hyphens: reinventing self and other in qualitative research. In *Handbook of qualitative research* (ed. N. K. Denzin and Y. Z. Lincoln). Sage Publications, California and London.

Fowler, J. (1981). *Stages of faith. The psychology of human development and the quest for meaning*. Harper and Row, San Francisco.

Frankl, V. (1976). Man's search for ultimate meaning. In *On the way to self-knowledge* (ed. J. Needleman and D. Lewis). Alfred A. Knopf, New York.

Frankl, V. (1992). *Man's search for meaning. An introduction to logotherapy.* Hodder and Stoughton, London.

Fraser, J. T. (1987). *Time the familiar stranger.* Thomson-Shore, USA.

Freedman, T. G. (1994). Social and cultural dimensions to hair loss in women treated for breast cancer. *Cancer Nursing* 17: 334–41.

Fromm, E. (1951). *The forgotten language: an introduction to the understanding of dreams, fairytales and myths.* Weidenfeld, New York.

Gadamer, H. G. (1978). *Truth and method.* Seabury Press, New York.

Geertz, C. (1973). *The interpretation of cultures.* Basic Books, New York.

Giddens, A. (1991). *Modernity and self identity. Self and society in the late modern age.* Polity Press, Cambridge.

Gilligan, C (1993). *In a different voice.* Harvard University Press.

Gillon, R. (1997). Imagination, literature, medical ethics and medical practice. *Journal of Medical Ethics* 23: 3–4.

Girard, R. (1986). *The scapegoat.* John Hopkins University Press.

Glover, H. (1984). Survival guilt in the Vietnam veteran. *Journal of Nervous and Mental Disease* 172: 393–7.

Goffman, E. (1971). *The presentation of self in everyday life.* Penguin, Harmondsworth.

Gray, R. E. and B. D. Doan (1990). Heroic self-healing and cancer: clinical issues for the health professionals. *Journal of Palliative Care* 6: 32–41.

Guba, E. G. and Y. S. Lincoln (1981). *Effective evaluation.* Jossey Bass, San Francisco.

Gunuratnam, J. (1997). Culture is not enough—a critique of multi-culturism in palliative care. In *Death gender and ethnicity* (ed. D. Field, J. Hockey and N. Small). Routledge, London.

Guntrip, H (1969). Religion in relation to personal integration. *British Journal of Medical Psychology* 42: 323–33.

Guntrip, H. (1971). *Psychoanalytic theory, therapy and the self.* Basic Books, New York.

Hampson, D (1996). On autonomy and heteronomy. In *Swallowing a fishbone? Feminist theologians debate Christianity* (ed. D. Hampson), Chapter 1. SPCK, London.

Hanh, T. N. (1991) *Helping the baby Buddha to be born.* The touching life transcripts Number 2, Leeds Network of Engaged Buddhists.

Hanh, T. N. (1993). Walking meditation. Call me by my true names. *The collected poems of Thich Nhat Hanh.* Parallel Press, Berkeley.

Hahn, T. N. (1996). *Living Buddha, Living Christ.* Rider, London.

Harding, M. E. (1955). *Woman's mysteries, ancient and modern.* Rider and Co., New York.

Hardy, J. (1987). *A psychology with a soul. Psychosynthesis in evolutionary context.* Arkana, London.

Harper, R. (1966). *Nostalgia: an existential exploration of longing and fulfilment in the modern age.* Western Reserve University Press, USA.

Harrison, J. and P. Maguire *et al.* (1995). Confiding in crisis: gender differences and patterns of confiding in cancer patients. *Social Science and Medicine* 41: 1255–60.

Hay, D. (1987). *Exploring inner space. Scientists and religious experience.* Mowbrays, London.

Hay, D. (1990). *Religious experience today: studying the facts.* Mowbrays, London.

Hay, D. and R. Nye (1998). *The spirit of the child.* Fount Publications, London.

Haight, R. (1979). *The experience and language of grace.* Gill and Macmillan, Dublin.

Heaney, J. J. (ed.) (1984). *Psyche and spirit: readings in psychology and religion*. Paulist Press, New York.

Heaney, S. (1996). *The redress of poetry, Oxford lectures*. Faber and Faber, London.

Heaven, C. M. and P. Maguire (1996). Training hospice nurses to elicit patient concerns. *Journal of Advanced Nursing* 23: 280–86.

Heidegger, M. (1962). *Being and time*. Blackwell, Oxford.

Heidegger, M. (1976). *The piety of thinking*. London University Press, Bloomington.

Herth, K. (1990). Fostering hope in terminally ill people. *Journal of Advanced Nursing* 15: 1250–9.

Higginson, I. J., Astin, P., and Dolan, S. (1998). Where do cancer patients die? Ten year trends in the place of death of cancer patients in England. *Palliative Medicine* 12: 353–66.

Higginson, I. J., Jarman, B. *et al.* (1999). Do social factors affect where cancer patients die? An analysis of ten years of cancer deaths in England. *Journal of Public Health Medicine* 21(1): 22–8.

Hillman, J. (1977). *Revisioning psychology*. Harper and Row, New York.

Hillman, J. (1978). Betrayal. *Loose ends*. Spring Publication, University of Dallas.

Hinton, J. (1994). Which patients with terminal cancer are admitted from home care? *Palliative Medicine* 8: 197–210.

Hockey, J. (1997). Women in grief: cultural representation and social practice. *Death gender and ethnicity* (ed. D. Field, J. Hockey and N. Small). Routledge, London.

Hockley, J. (1993). The concept of hope and the will to live. *Palliative Medicine* 7: 181–6.

Hoffman, E. (1992). *Visions of innocence: spiritual and inspirational experiences of childhood*. Shambhala, Boston.

Hoffmann, E. (1989). *Lost in translation—A life in a new language*, Minerva Publications, London.

Holden, T. (1980). Patiently speaking: motor neurone disease—patients' accounts of their illness. *Nursing Times* June 12th: 1035–6.

Hook, S. (ed.) (1962). *Religious experience and truth*. Oliver and Boyd, Edinburgh.

Husserl, E. (1962). Ideas: general introduction to pure phenomenology. Collier, New York.

Illich, I. (1973). The eloquence of silence. In *Celebration of awareness*, Chapter 4. Penguin, Harmondsworth.

Jacobi, I. (1967). *The way of individuation*. Harcourt Brace and World, New York.

James, W. (1902). *The varieties of religious experience. A study in human nature*. Longman, New York.

Jarrett, S. R., A. J. Ramirez et al. (1992). Measuring coping in breast cancer. *Journal of Psychometric Research* 36: 593–602.

Jasper, K. (1970). Boundary situations. In *Philosophy collected works: Volume 2* (ed. E. B. Ashton). University of Chicago Press.

Jaworski, A. (1993). *The power of silence. Social and pragmatic perspectives*. Sage Publications, London.

Jensen, V. (1973). *Communicative functions of silence*. ETC 30: 249–57.

Johnston, W. (1974). *Silent music: the science of meditation*. William Collins and Sons, London.

Jonker, G. (1997). Death gender and memory: remembering loss and burial as a migrant. In *Death gender and ethnicity* (ed. D. Field, J. Hockey and N. Small). Routledge, London.

Josselson, R. (1996a). *Ethics and process in the narrative study of lives.* Sage Publications, London.

Josselson, R. (1996b). *The space between us: exploring the dimensions of human relationships.* Sage Publications, London.

Jung, C. G. (1938). *Psychology and religion. Based on the Terry lectures delivered at Yale University.* Yale University Press, New Haven.

Jung, C. G. (1961). *Modern man in search of a soul.* RKP, London.

Jung, C. G. (ed.) (1964). *Man and his symbols.* Aldus Books, London.

Jung, C. G. (1965). *Memories dreams and reflections.* Vintage, New York.

Jung, C. G. (1996). The archetypes and the collective unconscious. Routledge, London.

Kearney, M. (1990). Spiritual pain. *The Way* 30: 47–54.

Kearney, M. (1992). Palliative medicine—just another speciality? *Palliative Medicine* 6: 39–46.

Kearney, M. (1996). Mortally wounded. Stories of soul pain, death and healing. Marino Books, Dublin.

Kearney, M. (2000). A place of healing. Working with suffering in living and dying. Oxford University Press.

Kellehear, A. (2000). Spirituality and palliative care: a model of needs. *Palliative Medicine* 14: 149–55.

Kemp, P. (1996). Ricoeur between Heidegger and Levinas: original affirmation and ethical injunction. In *Paul Ricoeur: the hermeneutics of action* (ed. R. Kearney). Sage Publications, London.

Kerr, F. (1986). *Theology after Wittgenstein.* Blackwell, Oxford.

Kierkegaard, S. (1968). *Sickness unto death.* Princeton University Press.

Klein, M. (1988). Our adult world and its roots in infancy. In *Envy and gratitude: 1946–1963.* (ed. M. Klein). Virago, London.

Kopp, S. (1992). *If you meet the Buddha on the road kill him.* Norton, New York.

Lakoff, G. and M. Johnson (1980). *Metaphors we live by.* University of Chicago Press, Chicago and London.

Lawrence, D. H. (1993). *The rainbow.* Everyman, London.

Lazarus, R. S. (1993). Coping theory and research: past present and future. *Psychosomatic Medicine* 3: 234–47.

Leonard, L. S. (1987). *On the way to the wedding.* Shambhala, London.

Lewis, C. S. (1982). *On stories and other essays in literature.* Harcourt Brace Jovanovitch, San Diego.

Lewis, I. M. (1971). *Ecstatic religion—an anthropological study of spirit possession and shamanism.* Penguin, Harmondsworth.

Llewelyn, J. (1995). *The geneology of ethics: Emmanuel Levinas.* Routledge, New York.

Lomsky-Feder, E. (1996). A woman studies war. Stranger in a man's world. In *Ethics and process in the narrative study of lives* (ed. R. Josselson). Sage Publications, London.

Lonergan, B. J. F. (1957). *Insight: a study of human understanding.* Longmans, London.

Longaker, C. (1997). *Facing death and finding hope. A guide to the emotional and spiritual care of the dying.* Century, London.

Louth, A. (1994). *Theology and spirituality.* SLG Press, Oxford.

Luke, H. (1987). *Old age. Journey into simplicity.* Parabola Books, New York.

Luke, H. (1989). *Dark wood to white rose*. Parabola Books, New York.

Lunn, L. (1996). Healing and dying: St Christopher's Hospice. *Health and Healing* 40: 1.

MacCuish, S., M. Patel *et al.* (ed.) (1998). *Walking with the Bhagavad Gita—freedom from grief and despair*. Life Foundation Publications, Bilston, West Midlands, UK.

McFague, S. (1983). *Metaphorical theology: models of God in religious language*. SCM Press, London.

McFague, S. (1993). *The body of God*. Fortress, Augsburg.

McGrath, P. (1999). Exploring spirituality through research: an important but challenging task. *Progress in Palliative Care* 7(1): 3–9.

MacInnes, E. (1996). *Light sitting in light. A Christian's experience in Zen*. Fount Paperbacks, London.

McNamara, J. (1983). *The power of compassion. Innocence and powerlessness as adversaries of the spiritual life*. Paulist Press, New Jersey.

Madras, R. E. (1995). How outsiders became subverters of Christendom. The Jew as quintessential stranger. In *Christianity and the stranger: historical essays* (ed. F. W. Nicholls). University of Florida.

Marshall C. and G. B. Rossman (1989). *Designing qualitative research*. Sage Publications, Newbury Park.

Mathieson, C. M. and S. J. Hendrikus (1995*a*). *Renegotiating identity: cancer narratives*. Blackwell, Oxford.

Mathieson, C. M. and S. J. Hendrikus (1995*b*). Renegotiation of identity: cancer narratives. *Sociology of Health and Illness* 17: 283–306.

May, R. (1972). *Power and innocence*. Norton, New York.

May, R., E. Engel *et al.* (ed.) (1950). *Existence*. Basic Books, New York.

Mayers, G. (1997). *Listen to the desert. Secrets of spiritual maturity from the desert fathers and mothers*. Burns and Oates, Kent.

Mayo, S. (1996). Symbol metaphor and story: the function of group art therapy in palliative care. *Palliative Medicine* 10: 209–16.

Metraux, A. (1959). *Voodoo in Haiti*. Andre Deutsch, London.

Merton, T. (1993). *Thoughts in solitude*. Burns and Oates, Kent.

Miller, M. E. (1996). Ethics and understanding through interrelationship. I and thou in dialogue. In *Ethics and process in the narrative study of Lives* (ed. R. Josselson). Sage Publications, London.

Millison, M. B. (1995). A review of the research in spiritual care and hospice. *The Hospice Journal* 10: 3–18.

Moore, T. (1996). *The re-enchantment of everyday life*. Harper Perennial, New York.

Morrison, R. (1994). Patients' sense of completion. *British Medical Journal* 308: 1722.

Moynihan, C., J. M. Bliss *et al.* (1998). Evaluation of adjuvant psychological therapy in patients with testicular cancer: randomised control trial. *British Medical Journal* 316: 429–35.

Murdoch, I. (1979). *A fairly honorouble defeat*. Chatto and Windus, London.

Murdoch, I. (1997). *Existentialists and mystics. Writings on philosophy and literature*. Chatto and Windus, London.

Neitz, M. J. and J. V. Spickard (1990). Steps towards a sociology of religious experience: the Theories of Mihaly Csikszmenthalyi and Alfred Schutz. *Sociological Analysis* 51: 15–33.

Nemo, P. (1985). Emmanuel Levinas: ethics and infinity. Conversations with Philippe Nemo. Duquesne University Press, Pittsburgh.

Nicholls, F. W. (ed.) (1995). *Christianity and the stranger. Historical essays.* University of South Florida.

Nouwen, H. J. (1977). *The wounded healer.* Doubleday and Co., New York

Nouwen, H. J. (1998). *Reaching out.* Fount Publications, London.

O'Connell Killen, P. (1997). *Finding our voices. Women wisdom and faith.* Crossroads, New York.

Ochberg, R. (1987). *Middle aged sons and the meaning of work.* UMI Research Press, Ann Arbor.

Ochberg, R. (1996). Interpreting life stories. In *Ethics and process in the narrative study of lives* (ed. R. Josselson). Sage Publications, London.

Payne, S., R. Hillier *et al.* (1996). Impact of witnessing death on hospice patients. *Social Science and Medicine* 43: 785–1794.

Perry, B. (1996). Influence of nurse gender on the use of silence touch and humour. *International Journal of Palliative Nursing* 2: 7–18.

Pfaffenberger, B. (1988). *Microcomputer applications in qualitative research.* Sage publications, London.

Picthall, M. (1953). *The meaning of the glorious Koran.* New American Library, New York.

Polanyi, M. (1958). *Personal knowledge, Towards a post critical philosophy.* Routledge and Kegan Paul, London.

Polanyi, M. (1966). *The tacit dimension.* Routledge and Kegan Paul, London.

Rahner, H. (1963). *Greek myths and Christian mystery.* Burns and Oates, London.

Rahner, K. (1966). The theology of symbol.In *Theological investigations IV.* Helicon Press, Baltimore.

Rahner, K. (1974). The experience of God today. In *Theological investigations II.* Darton, Longman and Todd, London.

Randall, F. and R. S. Downie (1988). *Palliative care ethics: a good companion.* Oxford Medical Publications.

Rees, E. (1992). *Christian symbols ancient roots,* Jessica Kingsley Publishers, London.

Reimer, J. C., B. Davies, *et al.* (1991). Palliative care. The nurses' role in helping families through the transition of 'fading away'. *Cancer Nursing* 14: 321–7.

Richards, T. J. and L. Richards (1993). Using computers in qualitative analysis. In *Handbook of qualitative analysis* (ed. N. Denzin and Y. Lincoln). Sage Publications, London.

Ricoeur, P. (1971). The model of the text: meaningful action considered as text. *Social Research* 38: 529–62.

Ricoeur, P. (1974). *The conflict of interpretations.* North Western University Press, Evanston.

Ricoeur, P. (1976). *Interpretation theory. Discourse and the surplus of meaning.* Texas Christian University Press, Fort Worth.

Ricoeur, P. (1978). *The rule of metaphor. Multi disciplinary studies of the creation of meaning in language.* Routledge and Kegan Paul, London.

Ricoeur, P. (1981). *Hermeneutics and the human sciences.* Cambridge University Press.

Ricoeur, P. (1984). *Time and narrative,* University of Chicago Press.

Ricoeur, P. (1992). *Oneself as another.* University of Chicago Press.

Rinpoche, S. (1992). *The Tibetan book of living and dying.* Rider Books, London.

Robinson, W. (1974). *Exploring silence.* SLG Press, Oxford.

Rogers, C. R. (1975). Personal thoughts on teaching and learning. *On becoming a person. A therapist's view of psychotherapy.* Constable, London.

Rogers, C. R. (1980). *A way of being.* Houghton Mifflin, Boston.

Roose-Evans, J. (1987). *Inner journey, outer journey. Finding a spiritual centre ineveryday life.* Rider, London.

Roose-Evans, J. (1994). *Passages of the soul. Ritual today.* Element Books.

Roy, D. J. (1994). During dying … a space for grace. *Journal of Palliative Care* 10: 3–4.

Roy, D. J. (1999). Why we need poets in palliative care. *Journal of Palliative Care* 15(3): 3–5

Rozin, P., L. Millman *et al.* (1986). Operation of the laws of sympathetic magic in disgust and other domains. *Journal of Personality and Social Psychology* 50: 703–12.

Salander, P., T. Bergenheim *et al.* (1996). The creation and protection of hope in patients with malignant brain tumours. *Social Science and Medicine* 42: 985–97.

Sapsford, R. and P. Abbott (1992). *Research methods for nurses and the caring professions.* Open University Press, Buckingham.

Saunders, C. (1986). *On saying yes.* St Christopher's Hospice, London.

Scannell, E. A. (1985). 'I've seen cancer from both sides now': an oncology clinical nurse specialist shares her own cancer experience. *Cancer Nursing* 8: 238–45.

Scarry, E. (1985). *The body in pain. The making and unmaking of the world.* Oxford University Press.

Schutz, A. (1964). The stranger. *Collected papers II: studies in social theory,* pp. 91–106. Martinus Nijhoff, The Hague.

Scott, P. A. (1997). Imagination in practice. *Journal of Medical Ethics.* 23: 45–50.

Seale, C. (1995). Heroic death. *Sociology* 29: 597–613.

Shipman, C., Levenson, R. and Gillam S. (2002) Discussion paper: psychosocial support for dying people. What can primary care trusts do? The King's Fund, London.

Silverman, D. (1994). *Interpreting qualitative data: methods for analysing talk, text and interaction.* Sage Publications, London.

Simmel, G. (1950). The stranger. In *The sociology of George Simmel* (ed. K.H. Wolff). Free Press, New York.

Skynner, R. A. C. (1976). The relationship of psychotherapy to sacred tradition. *On the way to self-knowledge.* (eds. J. Needleman and D. Lewis). Alfred A. Knopf, New York.

Smith, C. (1987). *The way of paradox. Spiritual life as taught by Meister Eckhart.* Darton Longman and Todd, London.

Soelle, D. (1975). *Suffering.* Fortress Press, Philadelphia.

Sontag, S. (1978). *Illness as metaphor.* Penguin, Harmondsworth.

Soskice, J. M. (1987). *Metaphor and religious language.* Clarendon Paperbacks, Oxford.

Soskice, J. M. (1996). Turning the symbols. In *Swallowing a fishbone. Feminist theologians debate Christianity* (ed. D. Hampson), Chapter 2. SPCK, London.

Speck, P. (1994). Working with dying people—on being good enough. *The unconscious at work: individual and organisational stress in the human services* (ed. A. Obholzer and V. Z. Roberts). Routledge, London.

Stein, M. (1983). *In midlife.* Spring Publications, Dallas.

Steindl-Rast, D. (1981). *Hanuman Foundation Newsletter* [Commentary] 2: 12.

Steiner, G. (1969). *The retreat from the word. Language and silence.* Penguin, Harmondsworth.

Steiner, G. (1989). *Real presences—is there anything in what we say?* Faber and Faber, London.

Steiner G. (1992). *Heidegger.* Fontana, London.

Stewart, W. (1996). *Imagery and symbolism in counselling.* Jessica Kingsley Publishers, London.

Stiles, M. K. (1990). The shining stranger. Nurse–family spiritual relationship. *Cancer Nursing* 13: 235–45.

Taylor, S. E. (1983). Adjustment to threatening events. A theory of cognitive adaptation. *American Psychologist* 38: 1161–78.

Taylor, S. E. (1989). *Positive illusions. Creative self-deception and the healthy mind.* Basic Books, New York.

Thomas, L. M. (1996). Embracing our suffering. A Vietnam veteran and Zen priest talks of how he lives with the daily reality of his suffering. *View* 7: 10–14.

Thomson, N. (1997). Masculinity and loss. In *Death gender and ethnicity* (ed. D. Field, J. Hockey and N. Small). Routledge, London.

Thorne, B. (2001). *Personal centred counselling: therapeutic and spiritual dimensions.* Whurr Publications, London.

Thundup, T. (1996). *The healing power of mind. Meditation for well-being and enlightenment.* Penguin Arkana, London.

Tillich, P. (1962). *The courage to be.* Collins, London.

Tillich, P. (1963). *The eternal now.* SCM Press, London.

Tillich, P. (1964a) *Systematic theology 3.* SCM Press, London.

Tillich, P. (1964b). *Theology of culture.* Oxford University Press.

Tillich, P. (1964c). *Systematic theology I.* University of Chicago Press.

Tolstoy, L. (1996). *The death of Ivan Illich.* Penguin, London.

Torrance, T. F. (ed.) (1980). *Belief in science and Christian life. The relevance of Micheal Polanyi's thought for Christian faith and life.* Handsel Press, Edinburgh.

Underhill, E. (1995). *Mysticism: the development of humankind's spiritual consciousness.* Bracken Books, London.

VandeCreek, L and L. Burton (ed.) (2001). A white paper. Professional chaplaincy—its role and importance in healthcare. *Omni: Journal of Spiritual and Religious Care* 55: .

Vanier, T. (1993). *Nick— man of the heart.* Gill and Macmillan, Dublin.

Vaughan, C. (1996). Teach me to hear mermaids singing. *British Medical Journal* 313: 565.

Waldenfels, B. (1996). The other and the foreign. In *Paul Ricoeur: the hermeneutics of action (ed.* R. Kearney). Sage Publications, London.

Ward, H. and J. Wild (1996). *Guard the chaos—finding meaning in change.* Darton Longman and Todd, London.

Warnke, G. (1987). *Gadamer: hermeutics, tradition and reason.* Polity Press, Cambridge.

Watts, A. (1985). *The way of Zen.* Penguin, Harmondsworth.

Webb, C. (1986). *Feminist practice in women's health care.* John Wiley and Sons, Chichester.

Weil, S. (1977). *Waiting on God: letters and essays.* Harper Collins, London.

Weisman, A. D. (1972). *On dying and denying: a psychological study of terminality.* Behavioural Publications, New York.

Weisman, M. D. and J. D. Wordon (1976). The existential plight in cancer: significance of the first 100 days. *International Journal of Psychiatric Medicine* 7: 1–13.

Welman, M. and P. Faber (1992). The dream in terminal illness: a Jungian formulation. *Journal of Analytical Psychology* 37: 61–8.

Wheelwright, J. H. (1981). *The death of a woman. How a life became complete.* St Martin's Press, New York.

White, V. (1960). *Soul and psyche.* Collins and Harville Press, London.

Wilber, K. (1996). *A brief history of everything.* Gill and Macmillan, Dublin.

Williams, M. (1996). Men and bereavement: a general hospice survey. *Newsletter of the National Association of Bereavement Services* 21: 9–11.

Williams, R. (1989). A protestant legacy: attitudes to death and illness among elderly Aberdonians. Clarendon Press, Oxford.

Winnicott, D. W. (1965*a*). *The capacity to be alone. Maturational processes and the facilitating environment. Studies in the theory of emotional development.* International Universities Press, Madison.

Winnicott, D. W. (1965*b*). *The family and individual development.* Tavistock Publications, London.

Winnicott, D. W. (1971). *Playing and reality.* Tavistock Publications, New York.

Wittgenstein, L. (1969). *Philosophical investigations.* Blackwell, Oxford.

Wittgenstein, L. (1979). *On certainty.* Blackwell, Oxford.

Wolff, K. H. (ed.) (1950). *The sociology of George Simmel.* Free Press of Glencoe.

Woodman, M. (1985). *The pregnant virgin. A process of psychological transformation.* Inner City Books, Toronto.

World Health Organization (1990). Cancer pain relief and palliative care. Technical report series 804. World Health Organization, Geneva.

Yaniv, H (1995). Sexuality of cancer patients—a palliative approach. *European Journal of Palliative Care* 2: 69–72.

Yeats, W. B. (1982). *Collected poems.* Macmillan, London,.

Young, M. and L. Cullen (1996). *A good death. Conversations with East Londoners.* Routledge, London.

Index